KU-221-940

CULTURAL PERSPECTIVES ON MENTAL WELLBEING

Spiritual Interpretations of
Symptoms in Medical Practice

DR NATALIE TOBERT

Foreword by Dr Michael Cornwall

WITHDRAWN
FROM LIBRARY

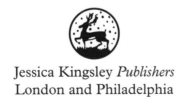

Jessica Kingsley *Publishers*
London and Philadelphia

Bullet list on pp.57–8 is reproduced with kind permission from Elois A. Berlin.

First published in 2017
by Jessica Kingsley Publishers
73 Collier Street
London N1 9BE, UK
and
400 Market Street, Suite 400
Philadelphia, PA 19106, USA

www.jkp.com

Copyright © Natalie Tobert 2017
Foreword copyright © Michael Cornwall 2017

All rights reserved. No part of this publication may be reproduced in any material form
(including photocopying, storing in any medium by electronic means or transmitting)
without the written permission of the copyright owner except in accordance with the
provisions of the law or under terms of a licence issued in the UK by the Copyright
Licensing Agency Ltd. www.cla.co.uk or in overseas territories by the relevant
reproduction rights organisation, for details see www.ifrro.org. Applications for the
copyright owner's written permission to reproduce any part of this publication should
be addressed to the publisher.

Warning: The doing of an unauthorised act in relation to a copyright work may result in
both a civil claim for damages and criminal prosecution.

Library of Congress Cataloging in Publication Data
A CIP catalog record for this book is available from the Library of Congress

British Library Cataloguing in Publication Data
A CIP catalogue record for this book is available from the British Library

ISBN 978 1 78592 084 4
eISBN 978 1 78450 345 1

Printed and bound in Great Britain

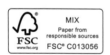

MIX
Paper from
responsible sources
FSC
www.fsc.org   FSC® C013056

CONTENTS

FOREWORD

The most memorable and operative sentence in this book for me is – 'Human beings are just starting to acknowledge that their frameworks of knowledge and beliefs about health are culturally determined.'

It is clear Natalie wants to hasten that exploration of the relative nature of consensual knowing and believing, especially in the hope of leaving the disease model of human emotional suffering and even madness behind. For her, she is part of ushering in a new paradigm that is more culturally universal – a paradigm that expands on the birthright of human nature to reclaim and embrace anomalous, psychic, shamanic, and spiritual experiences in a critically new way – a new way that prevents such intense experiences from being pathologized.

Natalie wants to accelerate what she calls the cultural u-turns that can happen when an out-dated paradigm fades and a new one surfaces and gains consensual favour – and brings the inevitable applications that affect huge populations once the u-turn has been sufficiently obtained.

The book's wide ranging table of contents shows the encyclopaedic scope of Natalie's field work and real world teaching, that informs her scholarship as a medical anthropologist.

Reading the book produces a very different subjective experience for the reader if one is used to wading through literature from fields of psychology, philosophy or religion/theology.

It's so rare to have a book in hand that addresses these three fields at once and more, by an author who is not a disciple of any one of them.

Like reading Gregory Bateson, one is left with the glad feeling of discovery that a first rate mind has synthesized multiple fields of study with the intent of shedding new light from an anthropological perspective.

I find such a wonderfully curious objectivity here that only arises when an anthropologist lens like Natalie's is keenly focused.

In other words, as a Jungian psychologist I gladly feel as if I'm unavoidably part of a myopic specialty profession that Natalie is kindly observing and taking field notes about!

As a practitioner and researcher of 35 years I'm refreshed to have me and my professional field itself researched by such an anthropologist as Natalie.

It's very valuable what she's doing in this book that is a reflection of decades of Natalie's real world quest to help us see the forest for the trees.

As Orwell said – 'To see what is in front of one's nose needs a constant struggle.' Or perhaps more elegantly put by Blake – 'The eye altering, alters all.'

Natalie may be both prescient and privy to hard won knowing when she asks and affirmatively answers this question that I hear from her in so many words from reading this book: 'Are we on the verge of a major shift in how health and especially mental health is understood and treated, that involves abandoning a reductionist disease based paradigm and embracing a holistic, open ended, even mystery filled vision of humankind – a vision that sees our universal need for the healing of our bodies, minds, emotions, hearts, souls and our inherent spiritual natures?'

Her answer obviously is yes.

I concur and would just add that seers like Jung and Joseph Campbell also saw a huge shift coming at even the mythic level, as the dominance of the patriarchal aeon looses its mythic power to hold us in its sway.

I'm grateful for Natalie's groundbreaking work here to inform and hasten the changes that may make life better for us all.

Michael Cornwall PhD

ACKNOWLEDGEMENTS

This book has a long history of inception, based on original course material I developed years ago when I transformed from being a quiet, behind-the-scenes anthropology museum curator to a front-of-house teacher of culture, spirituality and health.

Deep gratitude to those who first invited me to teach elements of the spirituality course, especially Bob Harris who introduced me to team-teaching, and Reverend Dorothy Nicholson who asked me to run a series of classes in her church.

Thanks are due to Fiona Bowie who, in the early days, had the insight for me to develop a course module on Rediscovering Spirit for her university students of religion and anthropology. I'd like to thank my tutors of medical anthropology who have passed over: Cecil Helman and Ronnie Frankenberg. While they were alive, each in their way was very supportive of my research into spiritual experiences.

Still very much on this earth is Elizabeth Archer, a former GP: we worked on a combined medicine and anthropology course, and practised team-teaching together in medical schools and hospitals. Her insights are included in this book on aspects of the body and midwifery. Thanks are due to the Alister Hardy Society for the Study of Spiritual Experience (AHSSSE), and to the Scientific and Medical Network, whose Blaker Education Fund supported the development of some of the training material on which this book is based.

I feel gratitude to the students of Brighton and Sussex Medical School where I taught for many years, and the hospital and clinical staff around the UK, who repeatedly encouraged me to write a book to support the teaching material. Particular thanks are due to Harjit Bansal who invited me to run courses as part of the Equality and Diversity Programme at North East London Foundation Trust. Comments from participants helped me understand what was needed for certain chapters, particularly those on death and dying. Thank you to Sarah Baxter and Shahram for their support.

Gratitude too to Natalie Watson, who kindly approached me, and invited me to submit a proposal: serendipity in action...thank you.

PREFACE

*Truth about human experiences appears to be culture bound,
time-specific, moveable and dependent on social consensus.*

I wrote this book to illustrate the systematic cultural U-turns which
occur in our civilization. The aim was to highlight the transient way
in which humans decide to follow a particular type of knowledge:
governments set laws regarding practice, and then we change our
minds about what is 'correct'. I wanted to explore the ephemeral
nature of knowledge and truth.

This book supports the medical anthropology seminar modules I
taught on Medicine Beyond Materialism courses, and it offers a long-
requested textbook to participants. The topics here are those I have
taught in hospitals, universities and medical schools, which throw
light on issues around cultural equality and diversity. The seminars
have been given in the UK, USA, India, Sweden and Switzerland.

On the one hand, I wanted to explore the extent to which ancient
wisdoms of originally remote societies were based on spiritual realities,
which westerners have long held 'in secret', and which are now
becoming popular and mainstream. But I also aspired towards raising
awareness of different ways of understanding health and interpreting
symptoms, so people might experience enhanced practitioner support,
particularly in the field of mental health.

In particular, two groups of people express dissatisfaction with
the current medical model of mental health diagnosis and treatment:
culturally new migrants, refugees and asylum seekers; and those who
have been within the mental health system (as service users, carers
or survivors), and perceive their condition to be part of a spiritual

emergency/emergence/awakening. Also there are psychiatrists who are aware their training doesn't fit the spirit of our times.

It seems as if there are several concurrent philosophies about human experience: one is visible on social media, of people who have been or are mental health service users, and are angry with the diagnosis and treatment they received. They perceive their condition to be part of a spiritual awakening and aspire towards more healing strategies for symptoms of distress or anomalous experiences. New migrants are often grateful for the support they receive, but it doesn't always fit with their cultural understandings of being human.

In contrast, in medical schools, students are being taught about the biological origin of mental diseases of the brain and their pharmaceutical chemical treatments. Medical students are rigorously taught about the predispositions of this or that ethnic group towards psychosis, without engaging with people's psychosocial history, trauma, environment, discrimination or forms of social oppression. To be indelicate, this may look to some people like racist educational beliefs.

The lay public are somewhere between these two extremes: some carers believe in the biological model of 'in the mind' and want the best medication for their relatives; while others want a more open dialogue and therapeutic approach towards healing. People seek a compromise.

I wrote this book to suggest new frameworks of understanding and interpreting unusual experiences which in the long term would reduce the distress of experients. As for me, I received an insight many years ago – that mental health and spiritual experiences were on a continuum. This book explores that continuum: it seems that some people have spontaneous experiences which stop. Specialists like shamans or clairvoyants seek out experiences and can switch them on and off. But those who have experiences that they cannot control, or who end up coming to the attention of psychiatrists, have no on/off switch. The phenomenology appears to be the same but the effects are different.

I wrote this book to gather evidence about cultural events which illustrate radical changes and challenges to the common consensus. My aspiration is to illustrate that cultural U-turns are frequent and normal and I anticipate another U-turn in our ways of understanding and addressing mental health and spiritual wellbeing in the near future.

PART ONE

INTRODUCTION

Common consensus is a temporary state. Consensus often appears to be the gold standard of civilization, by which societies make and agree decisions, and yet consensus is moveable and changeable – within cultures, between cultures and at different times in history. Societies systematically undertake cultural U-turns in medicine, health practices and philosophy. Knowledge and objectivity appear to be ephemeral. Knowledge can be compared to the shifting sands of truth and the ever-moving nature of consensual reality. The proposition is that common consensus is a temporary state, and in order to adapt to it, we practice cultural U-turns.

This book developed from ideas about cultural equalities courses which I taught to frontline medical and healthcare staff. For years, I facilitated a programme on topics about health and wellbeing. It became obvious each time I prepared a new seminar presentation that people changed their minds regularly. I would say: 'This is what people *here* do for health, but people *there* think differently, or earlier in history we used to have different beliefs ourselves'.

I realized that I needed to look more deeply into the nature of common consensus, specifically around human experiences, health and wellbeing. I wanted to explore the extent to which social, religious and community leaders achieved consensus and then radically changed their minds about it over time. There appeared to have been huge shifts in public understanding and awareness about human activities, experiences and behaviour. Also, there were profound policy changes at a state level regarding human health.

I wrote this book to gather evidence about events which illustrated changes and challenges to common consensus. I wanted to explore evidence of the radical cultural U-turns that occurred in the past and put forward the proposition that change and cultural U-turns were normal and were possible again in the future, particularly in the field of spiritual approaches to mental health, experiences and wellbeing. Each chapter has an overview of the content at the beginning and ends with a summary of the issues addressed.

I had to be explicit about the spiritual influences on health. I was aware that the term spirituality had a vast number of meanings, and I wanted to understand each meaning more clearly. I wanted medical and healthcare practitioners and their clients to have an opportunity to consider which aspects were relevant to them. With the importance of the Cultural Equalities Act in the UK and cultural diversity in the USA, it became imperative to have cultural humility so medical and healthcare providers could understand mental health and healing from their patients' perspectives, and not just work with western models.

CULTURAL U-TURNS AND MENTAL HEALTH

The base of evidence against old-fashioned psychiatry and western medicine is growing. The tipping point for change has already been reached. This means that people, including doctors and psychiatrists, are looking for other ways of understanding self and health, which is one of the key issues to address. The books mentioned below challenge the psychiatric 'bible' which is the Diagnostic and Statistical Manual of Mental Disorders (DSM); the theory of chemical imbalances; the biological causes of mental illness; and the efficacy and benefits of pharmaceutical medication.

My intention is to fill the gap by presenting ancient global cultural wisdoms about the human condition, as well as modern spiritual insights into life and death, the body, health and wellbeing. In particular, I present new ways of interpreting human experiences, mental health diagnoses and treatment strategies.

One UK psychiatrist, Joanna Moncrieff, has questioned the traditional view that psychiatric drugs target underlying diseases and has claimed that it was a fraud that they corrected chemical imbalances. She has suggested that we should examine the real nature of drugs to practise better psychiatry.

The social anthropologist, James Davies, has illustrated how scientific research has been manipulated to benefit pharmaceutical pockets. In his book *Cracked* (2013) he presented the way the DSM was created, without reference to scientific evidence. He interviewed the originators of the DSM, set out the human cost of pathologizing suffering and described how drugs were supported by mass marketing.

In the USA, Robert Whitaker and Lisa Cosgrove investigated how pharmaceutical money had corrupted the American Psychiatric Association in recent years. They documented how the psychiatric establishment had misled the American public about the biology of mental disorders, the validity of psychiatric diagnoses and the safety and efficacy of its drugs. They asked whether psychiatric drugs fix chemical imbalances in the brain, or whether they actually create imbalances.

A growing number of psychiatrists are aware of the dilemmas facing their profession and the UK mental health services. Phil Thomas emphasized the importance of context for understanding distress, of understanding a person's cultural, historical and social influences which gave meaning to their lives. He suggested psychiatrists move away from the biological origins of distress and its pharmacological treatments.

In my own book entitled *Spiritual Psychiatries* (2014), based on fieldwork in India, I explored spirituality and traditional medical and religious practices for mental wellbeing. The text provided a blueprint for improving the western understanding of mental health and the human condition. Using evidence from 40 personal interviews, I presented philosophies of medical practitioners, Hindu, Muslim and Christian clergy, mental health patients and clairvoyants. The book was an invitation to medical practitioners, educators and patients to open the door to more holistic strategies for psychiatric treatment.

This new book does not fit within the conventional academic categories. It covers existential thought and is extremely wide-ranging, presenting the human experience from life through health, to death and beyond. It presents material from a spiritual perspective. I am not writing from a particular religious or academic viewpoint, nor am I promoting any philosophy or any philosopher.

My aim is to acknowledge the dilemma of different frameworks of knowledge and bridge the gap between the perspectives of physicians and those of their patients. Human beings are just starting to acknowledge that their frameworks of knowledge and beliefs about health are culturally determined.

Part One explores the human being and health and presents changes in consensus and cultural U-turns which have already taken place.

Part Two explores death, anomalous experiences and mental health. They are together because people's beliefs about death and beyond usually influence their interpretation of mental health symptoms.

WHY CONSIDER THE TOPIC OF CHANGE?

As a society, we systematically change what we understand as 'normal' over time and space. This can be a problem for those mere humans who are judged on their actions and behaviour. Sometimes, what is normal in one geographical location is not considered normal in another. Often within the same geographical location, our understanding of what is normal changes with the passage of time.

Strategies for human health and healing at a governmental level change: there were times when common consensus dictated a particular morality and local authority and religious organizations responded accordingly. In today's era of openness, certain past official actions (such as removing new-born babies from unmarried mothers because they were the result of sex out of wedlock) now seem to us wholly inappropriate and require acknowledgement and forgiveness.

When we review current situations in the world, we find that, in the age of the internet, few things can be hidden and nothing can be unseen most of the time. In the UK, if the BBC doesn't cover a story, then it will be mentioned on Facebook or Twitter. Everyone has a smartphone with a camera to record evidence and then upload and share it immediately. If our peer-reviewed journals omit to publish certain research topics, then social media will. It is not ideal, but sometimes it seems as if our respected mainstream is playing 'catch-up'.

In spite of this, it is still possible to reinterpret the same event as truth or not truth and for culturally bound knowledge to dominate in certain fields of health. In the following chapters in Part One, I will explore the inconsistencies around the body and health from the perspective of medical anthropology and from western and non-western global ideas. I present consistent examples of cultural U-turns.

SUMMARY OF CONTENTS
Part One
Introduction

The introduction presents the structure of the book and sets out the key aim of exploring the changing face of common consensus over time and place. It explores our beliefs about the nature of reality itself, and the ways our interpretations of human experiences are modified over time. It introduces concepts around the cultural U-turn and culture-bound knowledge.

1. Consensual Reality, Spirituality and Religion

This chapter examines why we need to address spirituality and religion in health, not only with regard to new migrants, and African and Asian minority ethnic groups, but also with those people who hold spiritual views about reality. It presents a variety of meanings given to the term spirituality and its relevance to healthcare.

2. Culture, Nationality and Ethnicity

In this chapter, I explore human identity and define problems with certain terms: Black and Minority Ethnic (BME), Black, Asian and Minority Ethnic (BAME), Black, Asian and Minority Ethnic Refugee (BAMER), host population, nationality, migrants, mixed race, skin colour, race, made-in-Britain, generational differences, census categories and ethnicity. I look at changing responses to skin colour and ethnicity over the years and present material on the existential beliefs of medical and healthcare staff in the UK and the USA.

3. Cultural Beliefs about Health and Illness

This chapter addresses people's cultural theories of illness causation. It defines disease and illness from different perspectives: cultural, spiritual, mundane and esoteric. It looks at the role of prayer in healing and uses ethnographic case studies to illustrate beliefs about ecology and health. It sets out the importance that the belief systems of staff or patients have on the choice of treatment for illness.

4. The Human Body

This chapter examines the ways in which the body is adjusted: modifications to the human body and body parts may include breast augmentation or reduction, new hips, a new heart or heart valves, the modification of the lips and buttocks and of the genitals. I look at the cultural notion of biological 'male' and 'female' and people who experience a mismatch between their gender identity and their sex at birth. I present modifications considered to be 'normal' and changing attitudes.

5. Beliefs about Conception and Human Identity

The explanatory models about how conception comes about of different societies in the world are discussed. I consider what people believe make up a human being from the time of conception and birth and look at the role of midwifery for the dying and the new-born. The chapter presents cultural understandings of the role of divinity, or ancestors, in conception and offers a variety of ways for understanding human identity.

6. Women's Bodies and Human Behaviour

In this chapter, I explore the status and value of women and ways in which these may change and be culturally different in some communities: some people may consider behaviours outrageously wrong, while others consider them perfectly normal. I consider beliefs about ideal human behaviour and actual human behaviour that influence the relationship between men and women. I consider topics such as sex outside of marriage, illegitimacy, rape, female genital mutilation, control and different types of marriage.

7. Cultural U-Turns and Changing Responses to Consensus

Here I summarize how things have changed over time. Changing responses include: sex outside of marriage, adoption, abortion, children out of wedlock and stolen children. I discuss changes that have occurred regarding the treatment of women, diagnosis and the treatment of mental distress, pharmacology, prayer and attitudes towards assisted death. I observe how social, religious and community leaders achieve consensus, create laws and then radically change their minds about them over time.

INTRODUCTION

Part Two

8. Cultural Knowledge on Death and Dying

In this chapter I explore different societies' beliefs about death and dying, or passing over, and the ways these influence people's interpretation of their physical and mental wellbeing. I set out preferred treatment at the end of life, and explore concepts of meditation, mindfulness and the notion of living wills. I offer insight into the topic of sudden death and its effect on bereavement in the living.

9. Beliefs about Survival Beyond Death

I discuss cultural beliefs about what happens beyond death and include concepts of reincarnation, karma and dharma. I explore the linear model and cyclical model of different societies' beliefs about survival beyond death. I present case studies which illustrate how staff with the same or similar clinical training often had quite different views about reality, depending on their religion of origin or their personal spiritual beliefs. I look at the implications of the beliefs people hold, regarding the interpretation of symptoms, bereavement and grief.

10. Anomalous Experiences: A. Religious and Spiritual Experiences

Human beings have had and have valued religious experiences since time immemorial. In Chapter 10 I consider different terms and meanings of the term religious experiences and present the results of two research projects.

11. Anomalous Experiences: B. Near-Death Experiences (NDE), Out-of-Body Experiences (OBE), End-of-Life Experiences (ELE)

The aim of this chapter is to explore unusual human experiences that may occur to patients in a healthcare setting and the concept of expanded consciousness. These kinds of human experiences used to come under the umbrella of religious experiences but they are now studied within paranormal psychology.

» 21 «

12. Anomalous Experiences: C. Cultural Interpretations of Mental Health

In this chapter I look at different cultural beliefs about existential realities, the kinds of experiences human beings have and cultural responses to symptoms of mental health. I explore what is considered normal and present social interpretations of mental health, spirit possession, *djinn*, psychosis and schizophrenia. I use case study examples from my research in India and work doing mental health promotion with African and Asian new migrants in London.

13. Anomalous Experiences: D. Popular Uprisings and Spiritual Awakening

The question as to what is or isn't a mental health problem is possibly the most contentious in this book. I discuss the fissures developing between psychiatrists and psychologists and the anger of some mental health service users towards the system. I present examples of organizations in the UK and the USA which question the older mental health strategies.

14. Anomalous Experiences: E. Deliberate Shifts in Consciousness

I explore those human experiences which specialists deliberately seek and present what is understood by clairvoyance, mediumship, psychism and shamanism. These skills are said to be on a continuum from normal to anomalous to abnormal.

15. Why Address Cultural Understandings and Academic Fixity?

There is a fundamental paradigm divide between those people who maintain a materialist view on life and those who hold a spiritist perspective of existence. The chasm between these two opinions or beliefs influences how people interpret anomalous experiences, or whether indeed they refer to experiences as anomalous at all. What happens when our mental health academic education system is fixed within one paradigm of consensus? How does this influence student education and training for our medical and healthcare providers?

16. Acknowledging Dissonance as a Way Forward

This chapter explores in some detail the dissonance between mainstream academic studies and social media: one presents certain types of data about human experiences to observers, while the other presents data on the same experiences, but interprets it differently. I briefly cover a range of topics including: critical psychiatry, epigenetics and loss and the potential value of acknowledging cultural interpretations of experiences.

17. Towards Positive Change

I make a series of suggestions and recommendations towards negotiating positive change for human wellbeing. I explore strategies such as lobbying politicians and deans of medicine and healthcare to develop appropriate training to support change and social wellbeing.

1

CONSENSUAL REALITY, SPIRITUALITY AND RELIGION

For a while in history, in parts of the western world, common consensus decreed that the practice of medicine and health did not require any input from religion or spirituality. Apart from general physicians and family doctors, specialist medical doctors focused on ever narrower aspects of the human body. At the same time (since the eighteenth century), Indian and other homoeopathic practitioners continued to use a whole-person, open dialogue approach.

This chapter explores why spirituality is once again considered important for those working with medicine and healthcare. It considers the benefits of person-centred approaches when working with patients. It notes the importance of addressing religion and spirituality, particularly when working with people from migrant and refugee backgrounds. This is important because people's cultural understandings of the body and self may influence their access to healthcare or their coherence with treatment.

This chapter looks at the way we are in the world, our beliefs about existence and behaviour and the kinds of experiences some of us have, which might be interpreted as normal or anomalous. We consider the wisdom of several psychiatrists and physicians and look at the concept of mindfulness and the therapeutic relationship when addressing healthcare.

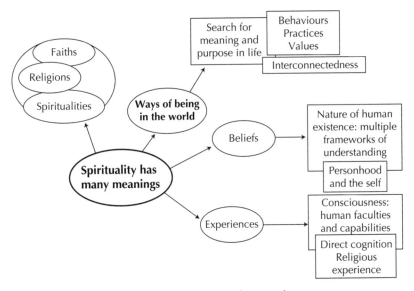

Figure 1.1. Meanings of Spirituality

WHY ADDRESS SPIRITUALITY?

What is the consensus about addressing spirituality? Within medicine and healthcare, once again it has become normal to address these issues with regard to patient care. Raising awareness of spiritual concerns allows us to: have an enhanced understanding of patients' religious and spiritual explanations for life events; support staff working with a client's beliefs; and, explore cultural presentations of symptoms. It also allows us to raise awareness of patients' beliefs, which may influence access to healthcare, and practitioners' beliefs, which may inhibit the kinds of treatments offered. Religion and spirituality appear to improve the quality of life for both staff and clients.

Spirituality has many meanings. It could mean our ways of being in the world: our search for meaning and purpose in life or our behaviours, such as mindfulness, good actions towards ourselves, others and the environment; or our practices such as prayer, devotion or listening; or our values such as compassion, conscience, integrity or our feelings of interconnectedness with others and the natural world. It could mean our beliefs about reality: about the nature of human existence, or our frameworks of understanding for personhood and the individual self. Finally, spirituality is also taken to mean human experiences: the nature of human consciousness, human faculties and capabilities; or religious experiences and direct cognition.

As well as spirituality, there are many cultural ways of understanding health, body and mind. Acknowledging cultural frameworks for the world and human existence is relevant to health and recovery. This is because a coherence of understanding between the healthcare practitioner and the patient tends to improve healing. When there is concordance of understanding between practitioner and client, due to increased cultural literacy about different models of life, there is a greater opportunity to encourage a significant response shift towards health and healing within the client.

Spirituality may be invoked in times of crisis or transformation, or when there is unexpected change, or in places of great hardship. It may also be invoked during great peace or in places of great beauty, or in times of transition during the life cycle: e.g. conception, birth, ill health, life events, death and dying, loss and bereavement, mental distress and unusual or anomalous experiences.

Religion is a more organized communal practice, usually within an institution, whereas spirituality is a more personal individual experience, which may or may not fit within an organized religion. Both may involve spiritual or mystical experiences, rituals, values, beliefs about morality and reality.

Religious practice usually has a cultural framework, with communal worship, a set of sacred truths and agreed practices. Those who practice have a reverence for a god or divinity or deities, and the rituals are intended as a means to connect with the divine aspect. There is an agreed concept of holiness and transcendence. Those who experience trauma or distress may feel they have taken a different pathway to 'being in the world'.

WAYS OF BEING IN THE WORLD
On being human and suffering

What is suffering? Viktor Frankl (1905–97) was an Austrian psychiatrist who was taken from Vienna to the concentration camp at Auschwitz where he spent three years as a prisoner of the Nazis. While there, he realized it was his fellow prisoners' will to find meaning in life and hope which motivated them to continue to exist. He wrote (2008, p.75): 'Everything can be taken from a man but one thing: the last of the human freedoms – to choose one's attitude in any given set of circumstances, to choose one's own way.' He survived the Holocaust and said 'the spiritual dimension cannot be ignored for it is what makes us human' (Frankl 1983).

Frankl suggested that if humans were in a situation where we were unable to change our circumstances (in cases of unavoidable suffering like Nazi concentration camps), then we could choose to change our attitude towards our condition. 'When we are no longer able to change a situation, we are challenged to change ourselves' (2008). He claimed that when the power of the human spirit is activated regarding challenging life situations, it can create a healing change. The last of the human freedoms, he said, was to choose one's attitude in any given set of circumstances.

NAZI PHYSICIANS AND ETHICS

During the Nazi era, in the concentration camps, physicians used human beings as guinea pigs in the name of medical practice. There was a different kind of morality to medicine in those circumstances. For example: 'Under the pretence of medicine, these doctors performed surgeries and countless experiments with no regard to the effects on the victims.'…'It was a watershed in the history of medical ethics and clearly a watershed in the history of human experimentation. These were physicians, of all people, who were involved in atrocities and murders. But they were all done under the egis of medical practice, under the egis of human experimentation that during times of war extreme measures require extreme actions. Physicians justified what they did by the need to get information…The physicians were in the position to make choices about who would and wouldn't be studied.'[1]

People who are ill want to make sense of their illness, and they may search for its meaning and purpose in their lives. When people fail to find meaning or purpose in their life, their will to live is weakened. A person's response shift towards healing seems to occur once they manage to change their evaluation of themselves (Sprangers and Schwartz 1999). Likewise, pain was said to be 'an unpleasant sensory experience' whereas suffering was 'a perceived threat to the integrity of the self' (Chapman and Gavrin 1993, p.6). A person's spiritual

---

1   https://weimarinflation.wordpress.com/secondary-sources

philosophy appeared to act as a buffer against suffering (Morgan 2003, p.112).

Therapeutic relationship and mindfulness

The therapeutic relationship was considered important, as was the amount of time a practitioner spent with a patient. At a health project run in Liverpool for chronic conditions, a person's wellbeing was an essential part of their considerations of the efficacy of a treatment, rather than the cure of their symptoms. The physician Larry Dossey (2001, p.29) has suggested the therapeutic relationship may be more important in the healing process and recovery than the difference between any treatments. The American psychiatrist, Arthur Kleinman (Kleinman, Eisenberg and Good1978; Kleinman1989), suggested that when practitioners listened to a patient's narrative, it helped them to understand how they made sense of their illness.

It has been said that the practice of mindfulness was also a very useful part of the therapeutic relationship (Kabat-Zinn 2005). Mindfulness involved a practitioner directing their attention to each experience, moment by moment, with open-mindedness and acceptance. They were trained to respond to whatever was happening 'in the moment'. Research on adults has demonstrated that those who learned and practised mindfulness experienced improvements in their psychological and physiological health. Evidence has suggested that mindfulness had positive effects on intellectual skills, improving sustained attention, visual-spatial memory, working memory and concentration.

There was also evidence from neuroscience: brain-imaging studies have shown that mindfulness meditation could alter the structure and function of the brain and produce greater blood-flow in areas associated with attention and emotional integration. There was increased grey-matter density in areas of the brain associated with learning, memory, self-awareness, compassion, introspection and reduced density in areas associated with anxiety and stress. Supporters of mindfulness meditation claimed it produced better and more effective leadership. Today, mindfulness is accepted throughout the western world as a useful strategy for frontline practitioners to work with their clients and for their own wellbeing.

Ignoring religion and faith

What happens in a secular society if we ignore religion and faith? The result of this may be negative. If certain groups feel they are being treated unfairly, they may cut themselves off and even work against that society. In 2015 the Mayor of London suggested we should not blame people of any faith for social unrest, nor should we blame British foreign policy. Meetings were held with religious and community leaders in an attempt to throw light on reasons for social unrest. The British Prime Minister and Mayor of London wanted to collaborate with community leaders to solve these kinds of problem, but each side appeared to interpret the situation from their own paradigm of understanding.

However, we may be courting problems in the West, if we consider it is normal to approach health and religion from a secular perspective. There could be problems if we believe religion can be reduced to a series of cultural rituals, sacred book and prayers. There may also be problems if we do not understand the deeper meanings found in religions and life, existence and divinity. The UNESCO Universal Declaration on Cultural Diversity claimed that 'cultural diversity is as necessary for humans as biodiversity is for nature' (Matsuura 2001, p.3).

SPIRITUAL DIMENSIONS
Beliefs about the nature of reality

I consider the topic of religion and health to be of great importance: research done for NHS Harrow and Mind in Harrow as part of a mental health promotion project with BAME groups indicated that religion and spirituality were key to understanding cultural beliefs about mental health (Tobert 2010a). The Department of Health published a report (2009) on the role of religions and faith in healthcare and was explicit about its benefits for mental health. The National Institute for Mental Health in England (NIMHE) project explored the role of spiritual beliefs in the assessment, support and recovery of mental health service users (NIMHE 2001). Research indicates that some disadvantaged groups are underserved within UK healthcare and there are disparities in access. We have seen that cultural differences influence health outcomes (Passi 2001).

Cultural differences lie particularly within beliefs about the nature of reality and the spiritual dimensions of existence. We have multiple frameworks of understanding regarding the following: the nature of human existence; the body and its faculties; personhood and the self; consciousness and survival after death; non-physical entities; and, the concept of life before birth and non-local mind. As this book progresses, it considers each of these topics in more detail. We know that the word spirituality has many meanings, but we do not seem to have any consensus about which ones we value.

Research illustrates that our frameworks of knowledge and belief influence our access to healthcare. In the case of mental health, people's beliefs about their existence influence their explanatory models for their symptoms and affect their access to healthcare and compliance with treatment.

Our beliefs about the nature of reality influence our thoughts about conception and birth: whether we assume conception only occurs as a result of a biological act or medical intervention, or whether we assume divinity has a role to play. Our cultural frameworks of knowledge influence whether we assume death is a full biological stop at the end of life, or whether we assume a model of consciousness after death, or hold some kind of notion of soul or spirit. It influences whether we accept the presence of ancestral spirits or earthbound ghosts. It influences whether we accept the notion of a good and bad death, or reincarnation and rebirth. Our beliefs influence our relationship with our body, and whether we consider that adjustments are appropriate for physical or emotional health.

MODELS OF REALITY: THEIR RELEVANCE FOR HEALTHCARE

Not only are there differences in cultural understandings, but there are also differences in people's beliefs about the nature of reality. Here are some examples: the earth is flat; the earth is round and at the centre of the universe; the sun sets and the moon rises; and, the earth is round and rotates. Today, common consensus only accepts the last of these examples as true – the other examples are assumed to be false beliefs of earlier times.

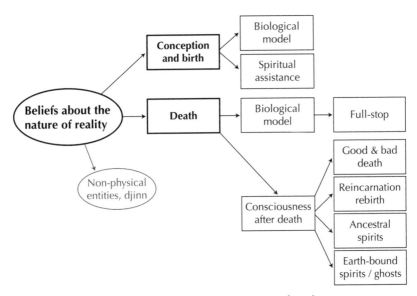

Figure 1.2. Beliefs about the Nature of Reality

There are some more examples concerning human life: you only live once; you are born, live a bit then die; you are born, live a bit then your body dies, but your soul survives then reincarnates (or goes to heaven or hell); babies can only be born from ancestral spirits; ghosts exist.

These beliefs tend to be considered cultural truths and their acceptance depends on a person's faith, intuitive skill or country of origin. Some say that all truth is culturally determined by majority consensus. This creates a complex problem as consensus tends to change over time and place and according to culture. Surely this must mean that the nature of truth changes? There is not one truth and one lie. Knowledge appears to be culturally determined.

The trouble is that it seems that there is no consensus as to what is knowledge. We would need to acknowledge a variety of different belief systems and negotiate a truth solution that fits each person.

Cultural blindness may exist: individuals in some organizations may believe cultural differences are of little importance; patients may be viewed through western cultural mainstream spectacles; and in healthcare organizations, subtle messages may be communicated non-verbally to staff and patients that their culture is of little consequence. In the UK, the Equality Act protects us from discrimination and two of the characteristics are 'race' and 'religion and belief'.

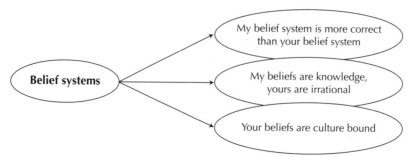

Figure 1.3. Culture-Bound Beliefs

NEGOTIATING BELIEF SYSTEMS

In what ways do we negotiate with the belief systems and the accepted paradigms of our colleagues and peers? A paradigm is a model or a pattern of reality. It is a set of assumptions, beliefs or opinions about how we understand our existence in the world. It has been said that paradigm blindness is the inability to see beyond one's own paradigm, which is intrinsic and therefore invisible. A simplistic view might be the commonly held assumption that my belief system is better than yours, my knowledge base is more correct than yours, or my beliefs are knowledge, whereas yours are culture bound. Simplistic, yes, but how much conflict is caused and how many wars are fought as a result of this assumption?

Scientific materialism is based on observable, rational and measurable physical phenomena which may be experienced through the accepted five senses. In contrast, the paradigm of consciousness and energy appears to illustrate the science of wholeness, interconnection and spirituality which includes and goes beyond physicality.

People's beliefs are important because they influence their access to healthcare. People's beliefs about their spiritual existence influence their explanatory models and interpretations of their mental health symptoms; they also affect their access to healthcare and compliance with treatment. It is important to integrate knowledge about faith and culture. Problems may occur if organizations focus only on religion (prayers, rituals and festivals) and do not engage with 'belief' when trying to adhere to the UK Equality Act 2010.

It is hoped that readers of this book will enjoy exploring the following chapters about cultural beliefs. It is also hoped that this may bring about an adjustment in their healthcare practices and support them in making future changes to their personal and professional practices. This may reduce practitioner burn-out.

SUMMARY

We have examined the topic of common consensus, its changing nature over history and the ways in which humans use common consensus as a gold standard of civilization to which society adheres by its rules. We have introduced social need, whereby we are either compelled to address changing morals or cling to them. We have explored why, as a society, we need to raise awareness of cultural diversity and people's subjective beliefs about the nature of reality.

This chapter has explored some reasons why spirituality is considered so important for those working within medicine and healthcare. It has discussed the benefits of person-centred approaches when working with patients. It has noted the importance of addressing religion and spirituality when offering medicine or healthcare to people with migrant and refugee backgrounds. This is important because data suggests that people's understandings of the body and self influence their access to healthcare and their acceptance of treatment.

We have looked at the ways humans are in the world, their beliefs about existence and behaviour. We have considered the wisdom of two psychiatrists, Viktor Frankel and Arthur Kleinman; their concepts of mindfulness and the therapeutic relationship are of critical importance when addressing patient-centred healthcare.

In the next chapter, I will introduce the delicate issue of culture and racism and the misunderstanding of 'foreign' ancestral origins, citizenship and Britishness in the UK and being American in the USA. I also consider the concepts of personal identity, ancestral origins, nationality, being foreign and ethnicity.

2

CULTURE, NATIONALITY AND ETHNICITY

When I am teaching, after exploring the different meanings of the term spirituality to enhance our understanding of human existence, the group I am with usually discusses what they understand by the terms culture and ethnicity. In theory the meanings are clear, but in practice we find ambiguities. In this chapter, I will thus explore the problems we have with certain terms in the UK: these include BME, BAME, BAMER, host population, nationality, migrants, asylums seekers, mixed race, skin colour, race, made in Britain, generational differences, census categories and ethnicity. In the USA there are other ambiguities; for example, who is the host population, who is a migrant and who are the original Native Americans or First Nations people? This chapter looks at the nature of objectivity and subjectivity regarding beliefs about human existence and identity.

CONSULTATION, COMPASSION AND EQUALITIES

When new patients come for a consultation, first, second and third generation migrants may look ethnically the same, may practise the same religion and wear the same style of clothing, but they may be quite different culturally and morally. For example, if we see two Somali female teenagers, we do not know whether one was made in Britain, with her whole history since birth in Britain, or whether she is a first generation migrant from Somalia or Somaliland who has seen and experienced unspeakable trauma. People of dual or mixed heritage, or who have parents of different religions, may have particular requirements regarding identity. There may be quite different models of understanding what it means to be a human being in different communities.

Compassion is essential within healthcare but it is not enough. Mindfulness is a practice which offers open-hearted awareness, focused in the present. It may help to humanize healthcare but it is not enough. These practices work effectively alongside cultural humility. Our aim is to understand and negotiate with a patient, combining their frameworks of knowledge with clinical models of health, to negotiate an agreement about diagnosis and treatment.

The problem is that subtle racism may exist within our assumptions about medicine and human beings. In many places it is important to consider culture, spirituality and health because there are so many different ways of understanding health, body and mind.

There is no longer one single truth. This insight was mentioned in Jeremy Paxman's interview with David Bowie. Bowie said of the 1970s that 'We felt that we were still living under the guise of a single and absolute created society where there were known truths and known lies, and there was no kind of duplicity or pluralism about the things that we believed in.' With the arrival of the internet it was shown that '[t]here were always two, three, four, or five sides to every question... The potential of what the internet is going to do to society (both good and bad) is unimaginable.'[1]

NATIONALITY

The multiple ways of understanding questions of nationality are explored below. I will address this because these are topics to which some people might assume they know the answer. Who is British – those who acquire citizenship, those who were born here? To what extent is skin colour and ethnicity assumed to be an indicator of Britishness? Is it the ability to speak the language, eat the food, have the appropriate hairstyle and clothing design?

For example, regarding the term 'host population', archaeological records tell us that African people lived in Britain as soldiers during Roman times (National Archives) and in the 1600s, during the Elizabethan period, there were graves of African individuals at

---

1   www.youtube.com/watch?v=YbeXIMhf8sI

Whitechapel in London (BBC News, 20 July 2012). Would we assume they and their descendants were foreigners or British?

British citizens have the right to live in the United Kingdom. They are those: of whom one or both parents are citizens; who are born in the country; who are naturalized at the discretion of the Home Secretary; who may be registered after five years' residence; or, who are adopted. National identity is a person's subjective sense of belonging to a place. Dual nationality is when a single person has a formal relationship with two separate countries.

British Nationals are those who live abroad and do not have the right to live in the UK. They are not British citizens. Sometimes we confuse nationality with ethnicity, culture and the ancestral family of a person's place of origin.

The word foreign has several definitions: belonging to another country; coming from a different country or simply unfamiliar. A stateless person is someone without nationality, citizenship or protection. An asylum seeker is someone who has left their home country for political reasons but whose claim has not yet been recognized.

The UK census monitors ethnicity; it records the ancestral origins of the population and their country of origin. In isolation, the data does not show who is first, second or third generation. The census does collect data on who was born in Britain or on new migrants from abroad. When patients present their symptoms at clinics, additional strategies are needed to communicate about their history and timeline of migration. Silence about past history or experiences of trauma or war may influence models of wellbeing and people's access to healthcare.

WHY ADDRESS CULTURAL BELIEFS?

Personally I find the census figures on religion and ethnicity that we collect in the UK rather confusing. It is not obvious what they mean. The US census has different kinds of ambiguities, such as over who is white or Latino. Using the UK census I began to explore the notion of identity: nationality, migration, culture and colour. In considering the notion of host and migrant populations, I would like to ask at what point and in which generation do the concepts of who is a host and who is a migrant become blurred?

In a country like the UK, 'western population' has a different meaning. Many people have migrated from other countries: there are first, second, third and fourth generations. At what point and after how many years do migrants become considered as the 'host population'? In the London borough in which I live, white people (whatever that means) make up 29% of the population, ethnic minorities make up 71%.

Research suggests cultural differences influence health outcomes. Ethnicity, nationality, race, religion, faith, culture and generational differences influence healthcare. Certain communities have negative experiences of healthcare or claim to experience inequalities. In the UK, some disadvantaged groups feel underserved by and experience disparities in access to the healthcare system.

Equalities

The Equality Act 2010 illustrates the government's position on anti-discrimination: if a healthcare or social care organization provides goods, facilities or services to the public, it must make sure it does what equality law says it must do. Equality law affects everyone responsible for running an organization, including staff or volunteers. It sets out the government's legislation on gender, race, disability, sexual orientation, ageism, religion and belief.

In 2012 Inservice Training and Educational Development (INSTED) produced a consultation paper on the government's legal framework and its implications for equalities legislation. Local authorities and schools had to carry out their specific duties to publish information about ways they were addressing diversity in January 2012, and from April 2012 they had a 'specific duty to publish measurable objectives'. They had to illustrate they understood anti-discrimination legislation, how different people would be affected by their activities and show how their services were 'appropriate and accessible to all' and met different people's needs. The Act covers all aspects of a local authority's work and its aim was to eliminate discrimination. INSTED suggested it was good practice to keep a record illustrating which equality duties had been reflected upon. This would ensure decision-makers undertook equality duties in a conscientious manner.

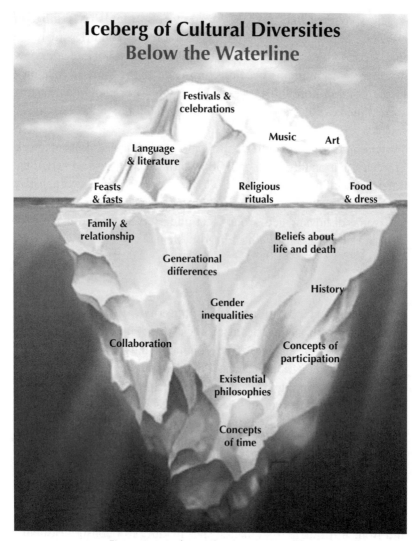

Figure 2.1. Iceberg of Cultural Diversities

However, the organizations responsible for equality and diversity appeared to change their names every so often: there was the NHS Equality and Diversity Council (EDC) and the NHS; then there was the Personal, Fair and Diverse (PFD) Council which was the new name for the EDC. Their aim was to embody the values and behaviours of the 'six Cs': care, compassion, competence, communication, courage and commitment. This was to be a vision to deliver: better health and better care; reduced inequalities; more accessible services; more clinically effective services; and, safer services with improved health and better patient experiences.

The World Health Organization claimed that there were a number of exclusionary factors to healthcare, including language and cultural values (Nygren-Krug 2001, p.6). They explained that our ways of understanding health and disease were part of belief systems which varied with each ethnic group. Certain individuals or groups tended to delay consultation due to their beliefs. The author suggested modern health service provision needed to account for different cultural beliefs in order to be sufficiently culturally sensitive so as not to limit the access of ethnic minorities.

Why address personal beliefs?

Our understanding of cultural diversity may be just the tip of the iceberg. We accept that it means understanding about religious celebrations and rituals, feasts and fasts, different languages and cultural literature and music and art.

These are all elements of cultural diversity but there are deeper aspects, as can be seen in the iceberg illustration in Figure 2.1. Furthermore, there are wide cultural differences between first, second and third generation migrants and people of dual heritage.

ETHNICITY AND PERSONAL IDENTITY

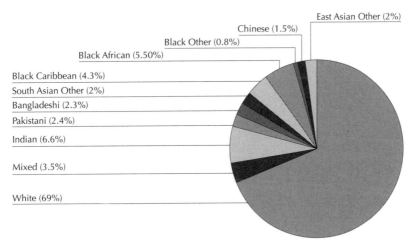

Figure 2.2. Ethnicities of London

UK census figures: what do they mean?

I want to examine what the UK census figures mean at a superficial level. Let us start by looking at census figures for one of the London boroughs: Barking and Dagenham. Figures 2.3 and 2.4 show the ethnicity figures for children on the school roll. White British are 39.6% of the population, White Other 9%, Indian 3%, Pakistani 4.9%, as are Bangladeshi. Asian Other make up 2.4% of the population, Black Caribbean 2.8%, Black African 22% and Black Other 2.1%. People of mixed race make up 6.8%.

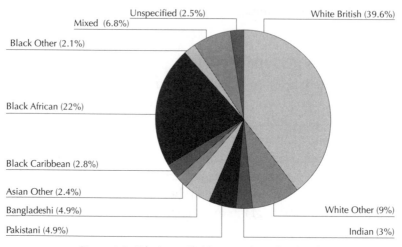

Figure 2.3. Ethnicity, Children on the School Roll

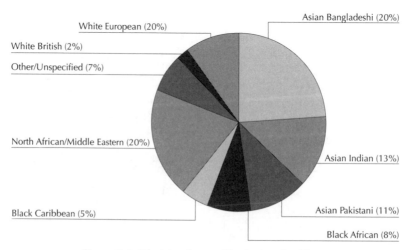

Figure 2.4. Ethnicity, Sports Charity London Tigers

A pie chart like this illustrates the ethnicity of the pupils' ancestors. However, the information needs to be expanded upon to illustrate the pupils' history and culture as well. Data about place of birth is collected by the government census. However, we cannot see from this simple pie chart which of the pupils is first generation, second generation or third generation. It is simply a snapshot of ancestral ethnicity. Some people are categorized according to colour, others according to place of ancestral origin.

When the ethnicity charts say Indian, what do they mean? The simple ones do not indicate religion: whether people are Hindu, Christian or Muslim Indian. Bangladeshi or Pakistani implies people of Muslim faith due to the partition of that region in August 1947.

What does Asian Other mean: Nepalese, Vietnamese or Burmese? Furthermore, I do not understand what the words 'white British' mean. Are they white British who have been in the country since the time of Jesus Christ or earlier? Are they ancient white British homo sapiens, Celtic, Roman, or are they third or fourth generation who migrated over the last hundred years, from Poland, Austria, Germany, Holland, Russia, Italy or Spain, to escape problems in the land of their ancestors' birth? At what point do they become 'the host population'?

Who are the White Others? Are they new immigrants from Poland, Africa, France, Germany, Romania and Bulgaria? Or are they new white immigrants from Iran, Iraq, Afghanistan, Jordan, Israel, Palestine, Turkey, North Africa or anywhere from the Near or Middle East? I felt it was unreasonable that the census of 2001 did not include people from the Near and Middle East, and I found it even more unusual that these people were not allocated an ethnicity category in the 2011 census.

Figure 2.4 was produced by the London Tigers, a sports charity originally set up to support young people in disadvantaged areas. Today it addresses employment, health, international issues and community cohesion. It is the only pie chart of ethnicity I have seen that includes people from North Africa and the Middle East (20% of the youth it works with). In the rest of Britain, people from North Africa and the Near and Middle East remain invisible in census data as White Other. Why, I wonder?

The census data from 2001 and 2011 appears to illustrate the ethnicity of the population's ancestors, based on skin colour and religion. If we do not acknowledge certain populations in the census, to what extent do we also ignore their presence as citizens and residents or patients?

BME, BAME, BAMER and host population

The abbreviations BME, BAME, BAMER appear to be indicative of a person's ancestral skin colour, place of ancestral origin, refugee status and ethnicity. I am not sure to what extent they accurately illustrate the culture or history of any of the BME/BAME/BAMER population. At what point in someone's migration history do they become culturally part of the 'host population'? Legally, when a person passes the Life in the UK Test, they can settle in the UK. However, when is a migrant not a migrant?

In Britain, it is a particularly tricky question to ask 'who are the host population?' Is it people who have been in Britain all their lives, and all their known ancestors' lives, or those who arrived ten years, 20 years, 30 years or 100 years ago? Or is it more to do with assimilation and integration? I also wonder what choices are made and what degree of assimilation and integration occurs. Is visual integration important regarding style of clothing, hairstyle, food preferences and agreed commonality of behaviour in public and official places?

I wonder if the invisible aspects of culture are also integrated; these might be beliefs about ancestors, ghosts, religion, the role of elders, the obligation of families, the behaviour of women or a preference for children of a particular gender. One's ancestors' skin colour, place of origin and ethnicity are interesting, but in medicine and healthcare it is equally important to understand a patient's or client's cultural beliefs and history whilst identifying their symptoms and strategies for treatment. It should be an integral part of medicine and healthcare to understand more profound aspects of a person's culture.

There are issues regarding clinical practice that require a deeper understanding of mental health symptoms: first generation migrants and refugees may hold belief systems about the meaning of their experiences and symptoms that are quite different from the those of the 'host culture' (a value-laden term in itself). Members may interpret their symptoms as requiring treatment from religious practitioners (e.g. church, temple or mosque) rather than from clinical practitioners.

This may delay people requesting help from mental health service practitioners. Therefore, it may be useful to suggest both clinical and religious health-seeking strategies to clients.

EXTRACT FROM *THE DAILY MAIL*

Walk into Ealing Hospital and you could be forgiven for thinking you were in a *foreign* land. Looking around the maternity unit, the vast majority of mothers with new-borns are from *abroad*. 80% of children born at Ealing Hospital in 2010 were to *foreign nationals*. Of the 3,289 children delivered, an extraordinary 2,655 babies were born to *non-British* mothers.

The statistics also showed that the maternity unit last year dealt with women from a total of 104 different *nationalities*. The children born to *foreign women* include 537 babies by Indian mothers, 389 Poles, 270 Sri Lankans, 260 Somalis, 200 Afghans and 208 Pakistanis. In contrast, there were 634 babies with *British mothers*, including just three from Wales and six from Scotland.

The revelations have inevitably sparked criticism of Britain's immigration policies, and renewed concern that the NHS is being overwhelmed by an influx of *foreign mothers* keen to take advantage of free healthcare.

And then there is overt racism. Journalism fanned the flames of racism at a maternity unity in North West London (Brennan 2011). An item was written for a popular national newspaper where the journalist misinterpreted the word 'foreign', and assumed every new mother whose ancestral origin was not 'white' English, Irish, Welsh or Scottish was foreign.

That hospital's new birth centre opened in May 2013 and it was the result of £301,000 investment in the maternity unit, but it closed again in July 2015. The issues broached in this piece of journalism call into question popular and professional understandings of national identity, being foreign, host population, Britishness and being white.

UK EQUALITY AND DIVERSITY

It is important to consider spirituality and health together; there are many different ways of understanding health, body and mind. Cultural knowledge frameworks for understanding the world and human existence are relevant for health and recovery. This is because a coherence of understanding between the healthcare practitioner and patient may improve healing. What practical steps might we take to open up the debate about faith and health? How might we support commissioning agents to make effective decisions about faith and health?

The NHS Equality Delivery System (EDS) was established in 2009, developed by the national NHS Equality and Diversity Council (EDC). It included Director Generals from the Department of Health and representatives from strategic health authorities. It supported NHS staff to work closely with communities to deliver fair services and promote good practice. It was part of a vision for delivering better health and better care, with reduced inequalities and more accessible services. The aim was to provide more clinically effective and safer services, leading to improved health and a better patient experience.

Central and Northwest London NHS Foundation Trust (CNWL) policy said that '[c]ultural competency involves an individual's ability to treat every person with dignity, respect and fairness, in a way that is sensitively responsive to differences and similarities, and thereby contributes to creating a genuinely inclusive culture'. For CNWL, cultural competency included: reflecting on and examining their own values, beliefs and cultural identity; understanding and challenging discrimination and racism; and, managing diversity as a routine aspect of clinical work and not as an exceptional event.

SUMMARY

I began this chapter by exploring the notion of compassion and equalities. I then presented the topics of nationality, migration, culture and colour by using the UK census. I noted anomalies in it regarding colour and omissions.

We explored the notion of host population and migrants and asked at what point in the multicultural western world and in which generation the concepts became blurred. We gave a brief overview of the changing world of cultural diversity and equality and the role of religion and spiritual beliefs in health.

When training was run for medical and healthcare providers, we found that although participants had similar training, they often had quite different beliefs about human existence. Existential beliefs about illness causation influence the way people interpret their symptoms and the way staff offer treatments for mental distress. Issues around racism must be tackled, but in the UK the Equalities Office appears to have its attention focused elsewhere.

3

CULTURAL BELIEFS ABOUT HEALTH AND ILLNESS

In the previous chapter I suggested that although compassion and mindfulness matter to ensure we do not make assumptions about a person or their health, culture and ethnicity are also important. This chapter describes a range of cultural theories about illness causation, from the mundane to the esoteric. Recently a lawyer told me that it is no longer appropriate to use the term 'black' when referring to the skin colour of people, but rather to use the identity of 'African'.

When I say cultural, I mean all of us. I don't mean any particular ethnic group. I mean all of us as human beings, in our geographical places, with or without religious or spiritual beliefs. Some case histories below will illustrate how we think about ill health and others how we change our minds about health.

I explore cultural theories of illness causation and popular beliefs about the body when it is sick and the variety of different cultural theories about illness causation held by medical and healthcare professionals and lay people. I start to define the concepts of disease, sickness and ill health.

Also presented are details from ethnographic case studies where sickness is linked to ecological wrong-doing or misdeeds towards one's ancestors. Although I mention theories of the causation of symptoms, because mental health is one area where there are many differences of opinion, I cover this in more detail in later chapters. I address the topic of psychosomatism, where different body parts may get sick, or where there is illness but no disease. The effects of prayer are mentioned, together with the role of religion in health and healing. Finally, I consider communication strategies, with the suggestion that those involved in healthcare might negotiate about treatment models until they find something that both the practitioner and client can accept.

RELIGION AND HEALTH

I often wondered what happened in earlier times and wanted to understand how health was addressed. In Ancient Greece, religion and medicine were linked; temples dedicated to the healer-god Asclepius were centres of medical advice, diagnosis and healing. On three marble tablets from 350 BC found in Epidaurus, the names, case histories, complaints and cures of over 60 sick patients who came to the temple are preserved. These patients slept in the sanctuary, near to the mineral springs. During their dreams, they were advised what to do to regain their health. This is similar to what I have seen in present day India, where mental health patients stay in or near religious buildings (Tobert 2014).

During the Roman Empire, the first Council of Nicaea was held in 325 CE and this urged the Church to provide for the poor and the sick: it ordered a hospital to be built in every cathedral town. At this time, the concept of reincarnation was suppressed. Then, during the Second Council of Constantinople in 553 CE, it was decreed that '... if anyone asserts the fabulous pre-existence of souls, and shall assert the monstrous restoration which follows from it: let him be anathema [excommunicated].'[1] This was an early attempt at controlling existential beliefs by making a law about life before birth and beyond death.

In India, religion and health were also linked, for example at Dharmastala, a Hindu pilgrimage site in Karnataka, where the temple trust provided hospitals, health services and a sanatorium for visitors of all faiths. This was replicated in medieval Europe, where some hospitals were attached to monasteries. In the UK, a patient's faith and religion were considered to be important to their wellbeing, and the Department of Health published a report on the role of religion and belief (DoH 2009). My own book on spiritual psychiatries provided data on the integration between religion and healthcare based on original fieldwork in India.

1   www.ccel.org/ccel/schaff/npnf214.xii.ix.html

SPIRITUALITY AND MEDICINE

We seem to have moveable definitions of what we mean by health and illness. According to the World Health Organization (WHO 1948), health is a state of complete physical, mental and social wellbeing and not merely the absence of disease. A state of illness is said to occur when the patient is aware something is wrong. Sickness is when that illness has been socially recognized and legitimized, either by a professional or by one's peers. Disease is the pathological entity.

Mental wellbeing is defined as a state of wellbeing in which every individual realizes his or her own potential, can cope with the normal stresses of life, can work productively and fruitfully and is able to make a contribution to her or his community.

Today there are many volumes written on the role of spirituality within healthcare. The American professor of medicine Puchalski suggested technological advances tended to change the focus of medicine from a caring model to a technological, cure-oriented model. Technology gave us the ability to prolong life. Until modern times, spirituality was linked with healthcare. Spiritual or compassionate care involved serving the whole person: the physical, emotional, social and spiritual. Patients valued compassionate care and the involvement of their physicians (Puchalski 2001). Koenig considered spirituality in patient care (2007).

However, I consider communication is as important as compass-ionate care. The aim is to understand and negotiate with a patient, combining their frameworks of knowledge with clinical models of health, in order to understand theories of illness causation and reach agreement about treatment. In that way, we acknowledge the different models of health and seek a healing strategy that conforms to both clinical practitioner and patient beliefs.

This is now the practice of Peer-Supported Open Dialogue, in which psychiatrist Tom Stockmann (2015) clearly presents the real changes occurring in the UK psychiatric and mental health system in the twenty-first century. He explains the Open Dialogue approach, which is a model of mental healthcare that involves a sufferer's family and social network.

CULTURAL BELIEFS ABOUT ILLNESS CAUSATION
Lay beliefs about illness causation

Medical and healthcare professionals may adhere to different theories about illness causation than lay people, and some may suppress cultural or spiritual beliefs they heard from their parents, grandparents or ancestors. Ideally, a mutual understanding between stakeholders would allow for an appropriate diagnosis to be negotiated and acknowledged, followed by the subsequent acceptance of treatment.

Mundane lay beliefs about the causes of illness include some of the following: risky personal behaviour such as smoking, drinking to excess, poor diet and other lifestyle factors such as sedentary living and too little exercise. Some people may believe illness is a result of mechanical or electrical failures in the body, or some kind of plumbing blockage – yet others suggest that stress, tension, anxiety and worry trigger ill health.

People believed they would be rewarded if they took proper care of themselves, ate the 'right' foods, exercised and behaved correctly. In contrast, they believed they would be punished by poor health if they did not take good care or behaved in an inappropriate manner. These beliefs about behaviour can be compared to those in Chapter 5 on the theories of causation for birth and conception.

In the past, western societies held negative beliefs or moral judgments about certain kinds of ill health, such as addiction, AIDS and cancer, or the ubiquitous belief that babies born out of wedlock were mentally deficient. Meanwhile, in other societies there were stronger beliefs that supernatural causes of ill health were of more importance, e.g. the position of the planets, the effect of karma, reincarnation carry-over, the evil eye, ancestral ghosts and *djinn*.

Toxins from environmental pollution are currently believed to cause harm to health, as is genetic inheritance and the expectation that diseases and family history will repeat themselves, so a person will be more likely to die from whatever their family members died from. Other popular theories of illness causation include the concept of impure blood: 'bad' relatives, being hot- or cold-blooded and having 'thin' blood.

Menstruation itself is considered differently, either positively as a sign of health and fertility, such as one's first period, or negatively as 'the curse', as unclean or polluting. For example, in Hindu temples women do not attend during their period: on or after the fifth day, they take a bath, wash their hair and then may attend. However, in Sikh temples, it was considered of less spiritual importance if a woman had her period.

The two case studies below are from Colombia in South America and Zambia in Africa. The first links illness to an ecological imbalance, whereas the second presents public open dialogue as a way to promote healing. The contemporary spirit of the times for looking at other cultures' notions of mental ill health is presented in the film *Crazywise*.

To make this film, Phil Borges and Kevin Tomlinson visited many societies in different countries and discovered each society had a shaman or a clairvoyant who acted as a healer to support others in the group (Borges 2015). These specialists were discovered by themselves having extreme experiences, which were recognized as symptoms of their gift. In Brazil, there is at least one psychiatrist who practises as a spiritist (Ramos 2014); she began seeing spirits when she was young, had a private practice as a psychiatrist and donated her time as a medium at a spiritist centre.

ECO-SYSTEMS AND HEALTH IN THE AMAZON

The anthropologist Gerardo Reichel-Dolmatoff (1912–94) conducted fieldwork amongst the Tukano peoples, living in the Amazon, in Colombia. Among those people, the concept of disease was closely related to environmental sustainability. The shamans were the societal healers. They believed sickness and ill health were a penalty which served as a mechanism to enforce rules about the ecology and the landscape. Illness was seen as 'the ecologically inadequate behaviour of the patient'.

Sickness was considered as a direct consequence of a person having upset the ecological balance. He or she was seen to have caused disease by their incorrect actions. In Tukano society, the shaman did not operate at an individual level. He or she worked to assess which part of the eco-system had been disturbed. The concepts surrounding ill health served to establish rules to address over-hunting, the depletion of plants and over-population.

The medical anthropologist Alberto Villoldo (2015) explains how 'psychosis' is a western interpretation of an extreme experience, and how we might learn more from societies which practise shamanism.

Other psychiatrists are becoming more interested in cultural theories of symptom causation, as well as the western biomedical model. The Canadian psychiatrist Joseph Polimeni (2012) made a suggestion that 'today's schizophrenia patients are no less than the modern manifestation of tribal shamans, people vital to the success of early human cultures'. His book was listed as 'highly recommended for anyone interested in mental illness or anthropology' in a review posted on the Royal College of Psychiatry's website, which has a special interest group (SIG) on transcultural psychiatry.

Another psychiatrist, this time in Russia, experienced a spiritual journey that she had not expected. Olga Kharitidi (1997) made a life-changing journey into Siberian shamanism which inducted her into ancient wisdoms. Her book is the story of her adventures in the Altai mountains of Siberia where she was taken as an apprentice by a shaman.

The reporter Anne Fadiman (2012) was instrumental in influencing change in American medical practice and education. Her book discusses a Vietnamese Hmong girl's medical treatment for epilepsy at Merced California and her local hospital's failure to recognize her family's deep-seated cultural beliefs.

Then *The New York Times* reported that a medical centre in California had developed a more cultural shamanic approach for its patients, a strategy directly influenced by research presented in that book (Brown 2009). A Hmong shaman performed a ceremony to summon a runaway soul. Under a new policy (the first of its kind), the medical centre recognized the role of traditional healers and invited the shaman to perform approved ceremonies.

There are many psychiatrists who are critical of their own institution's practices. Among them is Suman Fernando who challenged the orthodoxy of the dominant model of psychiatry. He explored the impact of colonial practices on global mental ill health, diagnosis and treatment. He claimed problems of living were becoming medicalized and overmedicated. He emphasized the importance of social triggers on ill health and was concerned about the denial of cultural and religious traditions.

Most seriously, he claimed the psychiatric system in the west was pervaded by an institutionalized or subtle racism, as outlined in his recent book *Mental Health Worldwide* (Fernando 2014).

In a similar vein, Ethan Watters is an American journalist who wrote about the spread of western culture-bound models of mental health. He claimed mental health was being Americanized by being exported globally across the world, to countries where it wasn't relevant. Below I present some examples of an African interpretation of mental health beliefs.

African interpretations and mental health

In a traditional African worldview, life is a cycle of birth, death and rebirth. This means that the spirit never dies; it is never destroyed only transformed. Although people can see their ancestors are no longer present in a physical body, many feel they can communicate with and act as spiritual guardians for their descendants. People revere their ancestors and may call on them in times of need. They maintain a relationship with them, and they act as spiritual guardians.

Rural Africans have different strategies for addressing suffering. After a traumatic event in Rwanda, people were uncomfortable with the western model of counselling which was offered one to one 'in a small dingy room'. Anthropologist Andrew Solomon (2015) said 'We had a lot of trouble with western mental health workers who came here immediately after the genocide and we had to ask some of them to leave.' In Africa, those who went to help assumed everyone addressed distress in accordance with western cultural norms.

PUBLIC HEALING IN AFRICA

In African countries there is a strong tradition of communication and public healing. The anthropologist Victor Turner (1967) conducted fieldwork with the Ndembu peoples of Zambia.

When Ndembu people became ill, their first explanation was that their ancestors had been disturbed by their behaviour. Sickness was also caused if a taboo was broken, or by quarrelling with kin. During a public ritual to release a man from troublesome ancestral beings, the participant recounted all his troubles aloud. It was like public psychotherapy.

During a public healing ceremony, it was socially acceptable for secret grudges and hidden animosities within the group to be voiced. A patient would not get better until all the villagers' tensions had been expressed or confessed. Speaking private matters in public allowed the angry spirit, which caused the sickness, a gateway to leave.

Turner suggested the purpose of healing rituals served to consolidate village unity, stabilize personal relationships and alleviate body pains and misfortune. In some ways the public healing ceremonies are similar to family therapy in the UK which emphasizes family relationships as important to psychological health. Those practising the therapy believe involving families directly often benefits clients and strengthens the wider social system.

The writer Malidoma Somé was born to the Dagara people in Burkina Faso, West Africa. He embodies a bridge between western and African ways of understanding and he has doctorates from French and American universities. He offers quite different insights into mental health. As he says: 'what those in the West view as mental illness, the Dagara people regard as "good news from the other world"' (1995). The person going through crisis has been chosen as a medium for a message to the community that needs to be communicated from the spirit realm.

Malidome Somé continues: 'Mental disorder, behavioral disorders of all kinds, signal the fact that two obviously incompatible energies have merged into the same field.' Disturbances result when a person does not get support to address his or her experiences. Alternative interpretations of 'anomalous' experiences, and ways these are addressed in social media, offer different models of health and mental wellbeing. As blogger Monica Cassani (2013) writes: 'The biggest problem in our society now for those who get diagnosed with any sort of "psychosis" is that they are most often met by professionals that do not even believe that healing can occur, let alone deep transformative growth.'

'In the shamanic view, mental illness signals "the birth of a healer"', explains Malidoma Somé. 'Thus, mental disorders are spiritual emergencies, spiritual crises, and need to be regarded as such to aid the healer in being born.' (Marohn 2014).

One man – Dick Russell – took his son, whom he said had schizophrenia, to see Malidoma Somé in Jamaica. The son had been in and out of hospital, had taken medication and put on a lot of weight. He wanted to contact Malidoma Somé because in his country of origin 'schizophrenics are not viewed pathologically, but often as mediums bringing messages to the community from the spirit world' (Russell 2015). In this case, African shamanic strategies were useful for addressing American schizophrenia-like events in this man's son. In a study by the World Health Organization, nearly two thirds of patients diagnosed with schizophrenia in countries like Nigeria and India had good outcomes, compared to 37% in the developed west (Barbato 1998, Haro *et al.* 2011).

THE EFFECT OF PRAYER ON SYMPTOMS AND HEALTH

Much discussion has taken place about the role of prayer in addressing serious symptoms. Patients and their relatives have used prayer and medical treatment for various clinical conditions at the same time. Prayers were said both for general wellness and for alleviating symptoms. Although people tended not to discuss prayer with their physicians, they did find it useful and believed in its healing powers (McCaffrey *et al.* 2004). As the American epidemiologist, Levin, has noted (2001, p.223): 'The weight of published evidence overwhelmingly confirms that our spiritual life influences our health. This can no longer be ignored.'

Intercessory prayer is done by one person on behalf of another. Scientific trials have been performed of intercessory prayer for heart patients at Duke University in the USA. The university reported that there was 'an intangible healing influence brought about without the use of a drug, device or surgical procedure' with 748 patients with coronary artery disease (Krucoff *et al.* 2005, p.216).

During the trials, researchers found distant prayer and the bedside use of Music, Imagery and Touch (MIT) therapy did not have a significant effect upon the primary clinical outcome observed in patients undergoing certain heart procedures. Therapeutic effects were noted, however, in secondary measures such as the emotional distress of patients, their re-hospitalization and death rates.

Dr Krucoff has noted there were many 'ancient healing modalities in all of the world's cultures'. He has suggested that 'the scientific literature and understanding of the role of intangible human capacities in our world of high-tech medical care' are 'very, very young'. Religious involvement was said to lead to lower blood pressure, fewer strokes and greater longevity. A list of early healthcare publications on prayer is available (Ehman 2006).

Prayer has been said to be 'one of the most prevalent forms of healing. Open-minded scientists have a responsibility to look into this.' Other responses from America include one from the *Washington Post* saying that 'prayer is the most common complement to mainstream medicine, far outpacing acupuncture, herbs, vitamins and other alternative remedies'. 'In churches, mosques, ashrams, "healing rooms," prayer groups and homes nationwide, millions of Americans offer prayers daily to heal themselves' (Stein 2006).

Religion and spirituality

In the UK, the Mental Health Foundation conducted a study on the impact of spirituality on mental health (Cornah 2006). They discovered that 'religion plays a central role in the processes of reconstructing a sense of self and recovery'. Some people found hope, meaning and comfort in their spiritual beliefs and religious practices (Cook *et al.* 2009).

The 2001 census of the UK population illustrated the following religious breakdown: there were approximately 42 million Christians, 1.5 million Muslims, over 500,000 Hindus, 340,000 Sikhs, over 250,000 Jews and many smaller religious communities. Findings have shown that a collaborative approach to religious coping (i.e. the individual collaborates with 'God' in coping with stress) was associated with the greatest improvement in mental health.

In 2012, Pope Benedict XVI announced that the Catholic Church was celebrating a Year of Faith from 11 October 2012 to 24 November 2013. He invited people to spend the coming year learning their faith better, living it more fully, reflecting on it and celebrating it together. The current pontiff has identified that medicine needs to heal the injuries of the sick before we ask about more mundane or spiritual aspects to health. In an interview with the magazine *America*, Pope Francis said: 'I see the church as a field hospital after battle. It is useless to ask a seriously injured person if he has high cholesterol and about the level of his blood sugars. You have to heal his wounds. Then we can talk about everything else.'[2]

---

2   http://americamagazine.org/pope-interview

PSYCHOSOMATIC ILLNESS

In some societies, illnesses are somatized. A psychosomatic illness is one which seems to have no organic cause, i.e. nothing biologically 'wrong' with the body or any of the organs. A person's emotions may be expressed by having 'something wrong' with the physical body. In some cultures, it may be far more acceptable to have a bodily illness than to have expressed emotional discomfort. This may occur particularly in the case of mental ill health which is far more stigmatizing than having physical distress.

Furthermore, some people separate their bodily disorders from their concept of 'self', whereas emotions tend to be easily linked to our 'selves'. In contrast, physical problems may seem more acceptable and can be separated from concept of 'self'. In some societies, there may be less stigma attached to bodily illness; it may be easier to say 'I have a pain' rather than 'I am anxious' or 'I am depressed'.

Studies have been developed to understand psychosomatic ill health from a holistic perspective, thereby throwing light on the relationship between biological, psychological and social phenomena. Psychosomatic disorders often had an unknown aetiology and they were unpredictable and less controllable than organic disorders: the patient's 'organ choice' could not be predicted.

In some societies, illness was a way of making explicit – in a culturally acceptable manner – that a person had experienced conflicts within their social, economic, political, environmental or supernatural relationships.

In the west, it has been the tradition that counsellors and therapists have tried to encourage their clients to express distress, during the prescribed timing of the sessions, in terms of psychology and emotions. However, other societies were less accustomed to this way of behaving. Unacknowledged stress due to external factors was said to manifest itself in various ways and may result in non-specific organ malfunction.

The psychiatrist Arthur Kleinman (*et al.* 1978) had an insight into the therapeutic interaction, which is only just being systematically incorporated into mainstream education for medical and health professions. He explained how clinical reality was viewed differently by the doctor and the patient and noted that 'systematic inattention to illness is in part responsible for patient non-compliance, patient and family dissatisfaction with professional healthcare, and inadequate clinical care'.

Kleinman went on to explain that disease and illness were separate elements of 'sickness'; disease was a malfunction of the biological system, whereas illness was a sufferer's experience and response to their symptoms. Today, the practice of Open Dialogue has taken on his suggestions regarding the therapeutic encounter and it is starting to reach into statutory healthcare.

COMMUNICATION AND NEGOTIATION ABOUT HEALTH

Doctors and patients may have very different notions of ill health and an ideal solution would be to develop communication strategies to address these differences and come up with a negotiated solution regarding treatment. The psychiatrist Arthur Kleinman developed eight questions which practitioners could use with their patients. Other practitioners like Bhui and Bhugra (2002a) have developed similar questions. Kleinman's questions are as follows:

- What do you think has caused your problem?

- Why do you think it started when it did?

- What do you think your sickness does to you? How does it work?

- How severe is your sickness? Will it have a short or long course?

- What kind of treatment do you think you should receive?

- What are the most important results you hope to receive from this treatment?

- What are the chief problems your sickness has caused for you?

- What do you fear most about your sickness?

Berlin and Fowkes (1983) created an even simpler model, entitled the LEARN Model:

- Listen to the patient's perception of the problem.

- Explain your perception of the problem.

- Acknowledge and discuss differences/ similarities.

- Recommend treatment.

- Negotiate treatment.

For many years, Kleinman's insights languished on library shelves inside academic papers, but a new strategy has emerged which incorporates his suggestions with the new training of Open Dialogue. Since the 1980s, Open Dialogue has been practised in Lapland. Open Dialogue became the psychiatric practice in Finland and the originators have offered various resources for wellbeing.

The results of research in Finland have demonstrated that this approach reduces hospitalization, the use of medication and relapse when compared to usual treatment strategies (Seikkula *et al.* 2006). Across the world, there is a great deal of interest in this strategy.

SUMMARY

This chapter has explored cultural theories of illness causation and popular beliefs about the way the body works when it is sick. It has defined concepts of disease, sickness and ill health according to medical and social models. It has looked at the relationship between religion and health and beliefs about the cultural causes of ill health.

There was a brief section on the effects of prayer on healing and the role of religion in health. Ethnographic case studies were cited where sickness was linked to ecological wrong-doing or ancestral displeasure, where healing rituals were open and public. It has addressed the topic of psychosomatism where different body parts became sick, or where there were cases of illness but no disease.

Finally, we have considered communication strategies, whereby medical and healthcare staff involved with patients, acknowledge that each may have different models of health. The suggestion was that they should discuss acceptable treatment, acknowledged which model they each believed in and agree on treatment strategies.

4

THE HUMAN BODY

What is normal?

According to whom, at what time in history

and in what geographical location?

WHAT IS NORMAL?

I started teaching seminars on the human body at medical schools in order to encourage students to understand differing cultural beliefs about health and the body. I have also taught in hospitals to support frontline clinical staff in gaining a deeper cultural knowledge about their patients' (and their own) belief systems.

The question of 'what is normal' is key in medical anthropology. One of the questions I want to explore in this chapter is: what is normal, according to whom, at what time in history and in what geographical location? At what point is deviation from an accepted norm abnormal or just culturally different? In medical statistics, 'normal' consists of a range of measurements under which a health condition is absent and above which it is likely to be present.

According to one dictionary, normal is defined as 'conforming to a standard; usual, typical, or expected'. However, this implies that 'normal' is accepted by common or social consensus. In the eyes of some – and possibly more controversially – a normal person is someone who is considered to be free of physical or mental disorders. On this subject, the psychotherapist Eric Maisel (2011) claims that '[t]his matter affects tens of millions of people annually; and affects everyone, really, since a person's mental model of "what is normal?" is tremendously influenced by how society and its institutions define "normal."'

Within medical anthropology, we are taught that our understanding of the body is usually culturally subjective. The western assumption that bodies can be researched in an objective manner appears to be culture bound, if it does not consider a person's history alongside their social environment. Although no one doubts the excellence of a biomedical approach to trauma and accident, differences of understanding create a dilemma between practitioners who offer treatment and sufferers who experience distress. There appear to be many ways of interpreting chronic ill health.

In this chapter I will look briefly at the 'normal body', the notion of biological male and female, those who are born hermaphrodite and those who decide to change their gender. I will also present lay models about how the body works and explanations for beliefs about where the boundaries of the body lie.

I examine cultural modifications sometimes made to a human body or body parts, such as breast augmentation and reduction, new hips, a new heart or heart valves and the modification of the lips and buttocks. In some geographical locations, parts of the body may be given a different value from other places in the world.

There are also mundane ways in which bodies are modified by different societies, such as spectacles, capped teeth or hearing aids. However, advances in medicine mean that people may have new lenses in their eyes, a new liver or even surgery to replace a whole face.

UNUSUAL BUT NORMAL BODIES...?
Ambiguous genitalia babies

Our understanding of the term normal may be ambiguous. In some new-borns, the genitals may make it difficult to identify the infant as male or female. In very rare instances, the physical appearance may be fully developed as the opposite of the child's genetic sex. For example, a genetic male may have developed the appearance of a normal female. If the process that causes foetal tissue to become 'male' or 'female' is disrupted, ambiguous genitalia can develop (Kaneshiro 2015).

In the rare condition of hermaphroditism, where tissues from ovaries and testicles are present, a child may have parts of both male and female genitals. This intersex condition is rare, where babies have testicles as well as a uterus and vagina. In the past, parents usually made a decision about whether to raise their child as male or female within the first few days of life.

In the 1950s, staff at Johns Hopkins University in America decided it was better to assign gender quickly so a child could be nurtured into its allocated gender. This advice became globally universal and gender reassignment surgery took place in those early days without a child's consent.

The cultural U-turn started in 1993 when the Intersex Society of America was set up to address the needs of people who felt they had been harmed by such treatment (Dreger n.d.). They offered a chart on the new paradigm for addressing intersex and they considered that 'intersex is neither a medical nor a social pathology'. Their ideal future was one where there was 'social acceptance of human diversity and an end to the idea that difference equals disease'. They stressed that being intersex was not a disease and it did not need medical treatment, unless a person requested and consented to it.

TWO SPIRIT PEOPLE

Among indigenous American civilizations, hermaphrodite people were called Two Spirit and held in high respect: the anthropologist Sue-Ellen Jacobs (1997) has explored how such people felt about themselves. They were considered as doubly blessed, having the spirit of both a man and a woman. They were not stigmatized but venerated and regarded as teachers. Californian anthropologists wrote in-depth about gender variations among Navajo people who allowed and accepted diversity (Williams and Johnson 2015). Changes in attitude occurred with the coming of Europeans with their concept of sin and homophobic beliefs.

Gender dysphoria is where a person experiences distress because they feel there is a mismatch between their biological sex and the gender identity given to them at birth. People in the public eye who have transitioned include the former soldier Chelsea Manning, the TV celebrity Caitlyn Jenner and the actress Laverne Cox. In the UK, there was recently a case in the BBC news of a young boy who had gender dysphoria. He felt trapped in his male body and was accepted by his parents, siblings and school to become a girl.

In Switzerland, a gentle documentary film about Christa Muth, entitled *Two Spirits*, premiered in 2012. It portrayed how she had lived and worked as a man with a high social status, but she had had gender dysphoria since she was child and she finally transitioned into a woman when she was 60 years old. She kept her job in human systems management at the university where she worked until she retired. The film follows her choices and journey to Bangkok for surgery (Périgaud 2012).

There appear to be multiple explanatory models for gender dysphoria: biological (e.g. genetics, hormones, chromosomes in the womb, unusual developments in an ovum, an atypical brain and insecticides which contain DDT and oestrogens) or psychological (e.g. unresolved childhood issues, a close mother-and-son relationship, separation issues). It was originally thought to be a psychiatric condition of a mental illness (defined in the DSM as 'gender dysphoria disorder').

Others believe it has spiritual causes, in the form of a spirit possession by a spirit of a different gender. Edith Fiore (1995) has cited one such case study and also suggests that where the veils between incarnations are thin, a person may have had the chosen gender in a previous existence. This belief is particularly prevalent in cases from South East Asia but it is clear from the psychiatrist Stevenson's research (1977) that it also occurs elsewhere. In his blog, Charles Tart (2011) presents a psychiatrist's overview of reincarnation beliefs in different cultures and religions.

If the people around those experiencing gender dysphoria are not supportive, this can result in feelings of isolation and suicide. Parents may mourn for the child they thought they had. People who don't feel they are either a boy or a girl are described as 'non-binary'. In the UK, around 1% of the British population may not conform to a specific gender. The Human Rights Act (1998) protects their privacy and dignity, while the Equality Act (2010) protects those in transition who are about to undergo change from discrimination. The NHS Choices website also offers advice.

Albinism in Africa

In Africa, being a human with albinism creates particular problems: Josephat Torner in Tanzania says that he and other albinos are not regarded as human beings. His parents were encouraged to kill him in the belief that albino babies were a curse. Albinos suffer from a genetic condition that deprives their skin, hair and eyes of melanin so they are vulnerable to sunlight and bright light. Many suffer poor eyesight and may get skin cancer. Today Torner is an activist, promoting the rights of albinos. He says the threat of violence is real as 'society doesn't see you as a human being'. Children are kidnapped and killed for their body parts which are used in charms (Mitchell 2015).

Since 2000, 72 Tanzanian albinos have been murdered, motivated by a trade in albino body parts which some believe have magical power. The government opened shelters specifically for albino children and commissioned a taskforce to investigate the killings. Some say that albinos are ghosts who are cursed, but by contrast their body parts are said to ward off bad luck and bring wealth and success.

Being born with albinism can be a death sentence in Tanzania and it has been claimed that the mutilation and murder of albino children have been met with social silence. The United Nations High Commissioner for Human Rights recently published a report on discrimination against people with albinism, and the Under the Same Sun activist, Peter Ash, aims to protect albinos from persecution.

Thalidomide babies

Children born with the effects of thalidomide also face certain problems. In 2008, a documentary called *Nobody's Perfect* was released (DW 2008). Using 11 people born after their mothers had taken thalidomide, the documentary maker asked them questions about their lives. People came from various backgrounds including politics, sport and acting. Each of them had accepted their condition and refused to let it stand in their way.

Thalidomide was developed by a German pharmaceutical company and was sold from 1957 to 1961 to combat morning sickness in pregnancy. There were catastrophic results for the babies of those who had taken the drug during pregnancy. As a result of its use, 10,000 babies were born with disabilities.

The Complete Marbles

In New York, the sculptor Marc Quinn exhibited a series of marble portraits of amputees and disabled people (2004). Although they appeared to be fragments, like the classical marbles at the British Museum, they were portraits of complete, whole people.

Quinn used 'imperfect' bodies to question the concept of 'perfection'. He said that each of the people he worked with had used their free will to overcome their biological realities, to become real-life heroes. That is why he wanted to celebrate them. In 2005, the white marble statue of the pregnant woman Alison Lapper rested on a plinth in Trafalgar Square, London.

The question of normal bodies depends on what is normal in the eyes of divine grace. When we look at adverts in glossy magazines and TV programmes, do we see the soul of a person through their eyes, whatever their body shape or shade? As the thirteenth-century Persian poet, Rumi, has said: 'Your body is woven from the light of heaven. Are you aware that its purity and swiftness is the envy of angels and its courage keeps even devils away?'

LAY BELIEFS
How does the body work?

Human beings have different beliefs about the human body and the ways in which it becomes ill. Popular and medical beliefs may differ, for example in terms of the way in which illness relates to: the inner structure or anatomy of the body; the way a body works, its physiology and function; and, its appearance, its correct size and shape and colour and the theories of illness causation. Beliefs about illness causation are influenced by our social and cultural backgrounds.

The popular perception of body image is very variable. Some people may have a poor understanding of the location and size of organs within the body. For others, there may be confusion about the terminology for certain body parts: for example, 'stomach' may be used to describe the whole abdomen; and people's perceptions of their organs may overemphasize the part of their body involved with disease or illness.

A healthy body is considered to be in full control of itself, whereas diseased organs or body parts may be perceived as alien, foreign, not part of one's self or out of control. The diseased part may be described as 'weak' or as 'letting me down', and the distribution of physical symptoms may differ from what is anatomically correct.

Some people use a plumbing model of physiology, imagining the body as a series of tubes, pipes and cavities which are connected to each other and to the body's orifices. In health this means that a clear flow of fluids, such as blood and urine, is desirable. They assume disease occurs as a result of 'blockage', resulting in the retention of toxins and impurities that 'poison' the system and need to be cleared out.

Others may envisage the body's physiology as a machine: as an internal combustion engine or as battery-driven. Machine metaphors include the heart as a pump, a nervous breakdown or the need for a battery recharge. Furthermore, in the same way that machines need fuel, human bodies require certain food and drink and tonics, supplements and other remedies to support them. Faulty parts are considered replaceable with spares like joints, pacemakers, heart valves and hearing aids.

Beliefs about body boundaries

In some societies a human being is believed to consist of both physical and non-physical components, some of which precede and survive death. But where do people believe our 'self' ends? Does it end at the boundaries of our skin? Does our concept of 'body' align with our concept of 'self'?

Many people believe our body and our self have invisible boundaries. There is the space around ourselves in which we tolerate proximity: once it is exceeded, penetration seems invasive. Intimate, personal, social and public spaces are located at different distances away from the body's skin.

Only members of the healing professions are allowed to invade our intimate and personal space. However, there are other cultural preferences: people from some BAME groups prefer only male professionals touch male patients, and female staff touch female patients. These preferences continue even after death.

In earlier times during a hospital stay, patients may have become dependent, losing control over time, space, their body, privacy and their choice of food. The anthropologist and psychiatrist Cecil Helman has claimed that during hospital healing rituals, a patient lost their personal identity and individuality. In the past, their pyjamas and dressing gown were sometimes the patient's own, and sometimes they were hospital property. As Helman has said, 'rituals provide a standardised way of explaining and controlling the unknown' (2000, p.165).

How are patients treated in hospital today? Hospital gowns were designed 100 years ago and covered and retained the privacy of a patient's front body, but could leave the patient exposed at the back. However, steps have been taken since 2010 to create a new, more dignified and modest gown, leaving patients feeling less vulnerable.

BODY PARTS
Replaceable body parts

It has become normal to replace body parts that are not working well (Norton 2007) or that are not compatible with our personal vision of self. Evidence exists from ancient Egyptian times of prosthesis and surgery (Nerlich *et al.* 2000).

In this section, I will give a brief overview of a few body parts that can be replaced, identify a few problems that have occurred and present some changes of opinion which have ensued.

Artificial hearts

Doctors from the Implantable Artificial Heart Project in Louisville, Kentucky have claimed that they have made 'the first completely self-contained implantable artificial heart that may allow patients more time at home, without wires or tubes piercing through their skin' (Polson and Mackovic 2006). They said that 'the hope is that by implanting this unit in patients who would otherwise die of heart failure, these patients may live longer and with a satisfactory quality of life'. Although the device itself worked, the human body did not necessarily accept it.

Hip replacements

Every year around 70,000 people undergo hip replacements. Traditional operations use a metal ball and plastic socket. In 2012, patients who received hip replacements were at the centre of a major health alert over concerns that they may be 'poisoning their bodies' due to hip replacements. Since the 1990s, metal-on-metal types have become more popular. Most hip replacements consist of cobalt and chromium alloys or titanium and reactions may occur: minute metal particles may leak into the blood, poisoning it; muscle and bone may be affected leaving patients in pain (Smith *et al.* 2012).

Breast implants

The cosmetic procedures industry has grown tremendously and was reportedly worth £3.6bn in 2015. However, it has been poorly regulated. For example, surgeons kept no records of which women had received Poly Implant Protheses (PIP) implants. Up until 2014, fillers used to plump up the skin and buttock implants were thought to have no medical purpose – the same was true of Botox injections. Surgery was carried out for cosmetic reasons, for example to reconstruct the breast(s) after surgery and as part of male to female sex reassignment surgery.

Due to the poor regulation of breast implant surgery, problems came to light in 2012. One woman paid £1000 to have her PIP implants removed after they had burst, leaving her in agony with silicone leaking into her lymph glands. She had originally undergone surgery in 2005 to enhance her breasts after having children. Around 40,000 British women had been given PIP implants which were filled with non-medical grade silicone and manufactured by the French company Poly Implant Prostheses.

The French businessman, Jean-Claude Mas, was arrested in connection with the global breast implant scandal. He was charged with causing involuntary bodily harm and aggravated fraud and was sentenced to four years in prison for fraud. The sale of faulty implants resulted in a health scare which affected around 300,000 women in 65 countries.

Cleavage-saving surgery

Ian Stuart Paterson, a breast cancer specialist who worked at NHS and private hospitals in the Midlands from 1994 until 2011, developed an experimental surgical technique for mastectomies. His colleagues had raised concerns about this in 2004 but he was not asked to stop until 2007 when a review identified that his experimental techniques required closer scrutiny. He had conducted surgery without using a biopsy and without checking for cancer beforehand. Nor had he gained informed consent.

Mr Paterson had not followed guidelines and the trust recalled over 550 patients who had had a mastectomy. He was suspended by the trust in 2011 and by the GMC in 2012. The usual statements were made: lessons have been learnt; there was a 'culture of negligence'; this was 'a tragic case'; there was a 'culture of silence', with staff afraid to blow the whistle; there is a completely new trust structure; we now audit our procedures; and, inevitably, this could never happen again.

Buttock implants

Buttock implants became fashionable as a beauty process for a short period until mostly women began dying from the procedure. In Venezuela, after 15 women with implants died, others went to surgeons to have them removed (BBC 2014).[1] Since 1969, people have tried to improve the shape of flat buttocks, sometimes involving complications and health risks.

In the past, implants were made of silicone gel, but after the controversy with breast implants, water-based implants were considered preferable. These did not cause lumps of infections. Surgeons then removed fat from one part of the body and injected it into the buttocks, but this process resulted in the injected fat being absorbed by the body. Stem cells are now combined with fat and injected under local anaesthesia. Mary Perdomo, who founded the No to Biopolymers, Yes to Life organization, died in 2013.

Body organs as a commodity

In cultural terms, people have different responses to accepting an organ. Transplants become, in some senses, a form of commoditization of body parts. In the UK, the National Health Service Organ Donation website provided the following figures for twelve months between 2011 and 2012; 3,960 organ transplants were carried out from 2,143 donors; and, 1,107 lives were saved and 2,846 patients' lives were dramatically improved. A further 3,521 people had their sight restored.

In the United States in 2012, there were over 14,000 organ donors (8143 from deceased donors and 5870 from living donors). The total number of transplants that took place was over 28,000. Only 3% were from Asian donors and less than 1% from indigenous American people.

In the USA, there were more than 118,000 people waiting for organ transplants in 2012: over 96,000 were waiting for kidneys, over for 15,000 livers and over 3,400 needed hearts. In 2012,

---

1   www.bbc.co.uk/news/health-27066675

6,115 patients died while waiting for organ transplants.[2] The figures suggested that people from different ethnicities had different beliefs about the body and its organs, and were more or less willing to accept a spare part.

One story hit the press in 2013 when a British Indian eight-year-old girl went into a Punjab hospital for a minor illness, was injected and died. Her family feared her organs would be removed during a post mortem. Others claim she died from a reaction to the injection. Although the trade in human organs has been outlawed in India since 1994, there are claims that it still flourished on the black market. It is estimated that around 2,000 human kidneys are sold each year.

Wealthy foreigners were said to drive demand, with poor or illiterate Indians willing to donate in return for high payments. There was an international trade in organs for transplant from impoverished people in developing countries to the wealthy. In New Delhi, black marketeers harvested kidneys from poor Indian labourers and used them for desperate foreigners. However, many people voluntarily offer their bodies or organs for donation.

Organ donation is considered appropriate by some ethnic groups and not others. For example, around 68 transplants were performed in the USA every day, but until recently Japan did only ten a year. In Japan, transplants can only be carried out from brainstem dead donors, and the under-15s cannot give consent.

The *Asian Times* claimed 'hundreds' of Japanese people were travelling to China for organ transplants, where donors used to come from prison morgues (McNeill and Coonan 2006). The sale of organs for transplants is illegal in China, but in spite of this the black market is flourishing. It is estimated that over 6000 prisoners are executed each year and it was normal to use their organs for transplants for others. However, Chinese people do hold the view that a person's body should be buried intact and this attitude persists among elders. Perhaps in the past prisoners were less valued as people?

Since the late 1990s, there have been 998 kidney transplants in Japan, but most were from living donors. The rest were from people who had brain death or whose heart had stopped. 'We do not approve of receiving organs from executed prisoners, but personally I can't simply disapprove of it... There are just too few donors in Japan'

---

2   www.liveonny.org/about-donation/data/#Data%20US1

(ibid.). In Japan in 1999, each transplant operation was reported in the news. Before 1999, people who needed transplants either went abroad or died. Most transplants in Japan involved living donors.

Body parts and consent

Why are humans so attached to body parts, even after death? In early 2013, the BBC ran a story about body parts from children that had been kept by police without consent. According to the Police and Criminal Evidence Act, it was legal for the police to retain body parts during investigations. However, during 2012 a national audit discovered that from the 1960s onwards, police forces had kept body parts from cases which were no longer under investigation.

This disturbed relatives with deceased offspring: 'I'd like to know the reasons behind them keeping them, especially in cases like my own where there was no criminal investigation, no suspicion.' As one mother explained: 'We didn't give any consent for any part of him to be kept. We assumed we'd buried our child whole' (Kelly and Hooper 2013). As a result of the audit, the police had to pay for almost 100 second funerals.

The previous year, in 2012, the British public discovered that body parts of soldiers killed in Afghanistan have been secretly retained by the Army. Over 50 items of human tissue should have gone to families for burial, but were kept by the Royal Military Police. The Ministry of Defence admitted material was retained without consent. There was evidence of the systematic abuse of rules which governed the handling of body parts when forensic investigations were carried out: 'These have been retained illegally for no good purpose and should have been buried with their owners' (Kelly and Hooper 2013).

REPATRIATION OF ANCIENT BONES

Museums in the UK have long had to address similar issues from excavated bones, and from human remains collected from research fieldtrips overseas. Within the discipline of archaeology, there has been considerable debate about the repatriation of human remains.

The legal status of indigenous human remains held in publicly funded museums and galleries has been debated and repatriation requests involved the return of excavated remains to their descendants for sacred safekeeping or reburial.

In 2001, a UK working group recommended the law be changed to allow for the repatriation of remains from national museums. Some secular curators condemned this as a threat to scientific research. Some UK museums had begun to return human remains in 1990s and the British Museum started to make returns recently.

Other museums are removing human remains from their collections, returning them to their countries of origin, often for reburial. They have the power to deaccession human remains in their collections under Section 47 of the Human Tissue Act 2004.

Australian Aboriginals, New Zealand Maoris and Native Americans felt strongly that their ancestral remains should not be in museums. In Australia there was a code of ethics that recognized indigenous custodial rights over human remains. In America, repatriation is governed by both state and federal laws (e.g. the Native American Grave Protection and Repatriation Act 1990).

The Museum of London currently holds approximately 17,000 human skeletons excavated from the City and Greater London sites. An additional 65 skeletons or parts thereof are accessioned to their core collections. The majority are covered by Home Office licences from the Ministry of Justice.

These licences permit the analysis, research and long-term curation of the bones. Sometimes a licence may specify a reburial is required. Human remains are cared for by the Department of Archaeological Collections and Archive, Centre for Human Bioarchaeology and Collections Care.

SUMMARY

This chapter has explored the concept of normality and the body. I have looked briefly at the notion of biological male and biological female and have considered people who were born with ambiguous genitalia and those who decided to transition. I have included the way albinism was regarded in certain countries, in particular in Africa, and have presented the concept of the disabled body.

I have provided an overview of lay models and beliefs about how the human body works, and have explored cultural beliefs about where the boundaries of the body lie. Cultural modifications made to a human body or body parts have been examined, such as breast augmentation and reduction, new hips, new heart or heart valves, modification of lips and buttocks. Modification of genitals is addressed in the chapter on women and wellbeing. I have looked at the emotional attachment people may have to the body parts of loved ones, for example when they have been retained for research or observation and not buried with the rest of the body. The concept of normal is changeable and depends on personal perception, the historical place and time, geographical location and an individual's religion.

In the next chapter, I will present cultural theories of conception and people's explanations around pregnancy, the new-born and midwifery.

5

BELIEFS ABOUT CONCEPTION AND HUMAN IDENTITY

WHAT MAKES UP A HUMAN BEING?

In the previous chapter, we have seen that the term 'normal' can be expanded and its meaning depends on subjective personal beliefs. In this chapter, I will explore beliefs about what a human being consists of and look at the concept of personhood and self and the nature of human identity.

I will use examples from the ethnographic literature to present a variety of beliefs about being a human being and there are many different explanations for how conception occurs. Some societies believe humans consist of both physical and non-physical components, some of which both precede and survive death. I will present cultural understandings of non-physical elements of a human body.

Cultural beliefs about being born free

The data in this section throws light on some underlying assumptions about western beliefs about human identity. It presents cultural explanatory models for spiritual and religious influences on conception. In the past, we tended to accept that – as humans – we were born free and started life with a clean state. However, with the examples given below about babies, identity and the soul, there was a plurality of influences: on conception itself, on the unborn and on the newly born child.

In which case, one may ask: according to whose cultural beliefs are we born free? Born free with a clean slate seemed to be the almost exclusive belief of western populations, with the complexities of original sin being a Christian tradition and *yetza hara*, the original inclination of Jewish babies to violate the word of God and turn towards selfish gratification, which could be modified by prayer.

Personal identity and self

The issues are complex but the variables of belief about what exactly makes up a human being vary widely across cultures. In London I regularly facilitated seminars with frontline medical and healthcare practitioners (Tobert 2010a, b). Participants all had the same or similar clinical training, but when asked what they believed a human being was made of, they were surprised to find they often had very different religious or cultural beliefs.

In some societies, a human being is believed to consist of both physical and non-physical components, some of which precede and survive death. Not everyone in the world or even in the United Kingdom and the USA has the same beliefs about what it means to be human. People believed humans were made up of different constituents. For some, the self and the identity were fixed at the boundaries of an individual's skin. For others, the self included those of the same gender, the same religion, the same village, town or country. Our beliefs about transpersonal approaches to human existence appear to have implications for healthcare, particularly in the field of medicine and mental health (Tobert 2014).

There are many cultural frameworks of belief, knowledge and understanding. In the past, according to the medical anthropologist Byron Good, the population's underlying (perhaps arrogant) assumption was: my knowledge is better/superior/more accurate than your beliefs (1994).

Today, we understand that some people agree that humans were born, lived for a bit on earth and then died. Others believed that when we died some aspect of the self went to heaven or hell (or purgatory), or that some aspect became an ancestral spirit or merged with God. Each person appeared to have quite different beliefs about what happened after death. There didn't seem to be any consensus.

Ancient beliefs?

In olden times, the ancient Egyptians believed we went on to some other place after death. Ancient Peruvians, meanwhile, believed that an aspect of the self stayed here on earth after death, so bodies were mummified and buried with gold and silver coins. Hindus believed that a spirit went to some other level of consciousness and was reincarnated, either within the same family or in completely different families. The Inca believed the soul went to a place to rest, after which it jumped into a womb again when it was ready to be reborn.

I have looked at the ethnographic literature published by anthropologists in order to discover more about people's spiritual beliefs about personal identity and the body. Whilst in the western world some people were not aware of or denied existential realities, other societies were more explicit about their spiritual realities.

For example, anthropologists who visited Melanesia discovered that the Lelet people had elaborate beliefs about the human self (Eves 1998). They considered that human consciousness and the body were inseparable: a person existed only if both consciousness and body were united. The life force gave a person their capacity to experience, perceive and communicate.

A person was also believed to be the composite of all its relationships with others: those who had nurtured it or had social relationships with it. Once a person died, the body decomposed, the life force permanently separated from the body via the fontanel. It no longer participated in affairs of the living, although its presence could be invoked. A person's life force stayed around the burial place for a short time after death. It was not considered immaterial: it could be seen after death but during life it was invisible.

Life, birth and death were enmeshed. To the Lelet, a good death meant the 'form' (ghost or entity) was helpful to humans. In contrast: with an unnatural or premature death, the 'form' was capricious and dangerous to humans. They believed people who encountered ghostly 'forms' could suffer shaking fits and violent headaches, and children could fall ill or have disturbed sleep.

The preoccupation with soul and spirit was ubiquitous. Our understanding of the ancient Mayan concept of the soul comes from hieroglyphs depicting words and images on buildings and in tombs. It has been interpreted and correlated by anthropologists with present-day Mayan beliefs.

Ancient Maya occupied an area of present-day Mexico and the Mayan temples were used as gateways to the spirit world (Friedel *et al.* 1993). The human soul was considered to be eternal. Lineage shrines at sacred places by springs or mountain tops were 'sleeping houses' for souls of dead ancestors. When a person died, their soul stayed around for a while and then returned to the soul pool and into the care of the ancestral gods. A pregnant woman would visit these shrines so a soul could be planted into her womb from the ancestral pool. People believed a person's soul could move around outside the body during sleep, but specialists like shamans could intend their souls to travel out-of-body at will.

In order to explore the nature of the self, a symposium was held at Imperial College London (2009) with various physicians, including critical care doctor Sam Parnia and psychiatrist Peter Fenwick. Today's physicians have become much more interested in the relationship between the self, consciousness and death. However, it seemed that globally, in many non-industrialized societies, there had long been an interest in subtle aspects of a person.

Personal identity, self and death

In many societies, beliefs about death are intertwined with beliefs about birth which can only occur because, as we have seen above, an ancestor is regenerated into the foetus. The anthropologist Malinowski undertook fieldwork amongst the Trobriand islanders of Papua New Guinea (1929, p.145). He had to learn about reincarnation before he could speak about conception. He had to present biological and spiritual ideas together. According to the islanders, new life begins with death. Spirits of the dead are considered to be the only source of new life and they always return to people of the same clan.

Similar beliefs have also been recorded during the 1990s in Northern Alberta, Canada by the Dene Tha who consider themselves Roman Catholic (Goulet 1994). In each case, the identity of a new child is linked with the death and regeneration of an ancestor: sexual intercourse is considered essential, but not enough, for procreation.

In Micronesia among the Sabarl, new mothers wore the same dress as widows who mourned the death of their husbands: one ushered in a new physical birth, the other oversaw the birth of a new ancestor (Battaglia 1990, p.44). Among the Laboya weavers of Indonesia, pregnant women were considered to be containers of ancestral breath and temporarily in touch with the 'realm of the dead' (Geirnaert-Martin 1992).

CULTURAL BELIEFS ABOUT CONCEPTION

The above illustrates how the concepts of birth, life and death can become entangled once we look away from western reductionist assumptions about conception. People have different beliefs about what makes up a human being and about what causes a baby to be conceived.

The aim below is to present a few cultural explanations for conception. I also present a brief summary of eighteenth- and nineteenth-century midwifery to illustrate the history of cultural U-turns on changing responses to giving birth.

How are babies made?

There are many cultural explanations for conception which results in a baby. Amongst these, the most commonly agreed in the west is that conception occurs as a result of a sexual act between human beings of different genders. This is just one explanation and it is a universal western assumption. If we invoke spirituality and culture, we need to consider not only the biological function of a sperm cell from a male and an egg from a female reproductive organ, but also a multitude of other cultural influences on conception. However, even with western consensus among peer groups, we agree that biological sexual intercourse between human beings of different genders is not the only way to conceive.

There are many artificial reproductive technologies like in vitro fertilization (IVF) and other assisted reproductive technologies that can be used to enhance conception. In some cases, by using Artificial Reproductive Technologies (ART) a mother may feel reduced to the passive carrier of the baby. Her eggs may be 'ripened', then 'harvested' and 'fertilized' in a laboratory, before being 'implanted' in a pre-prepared uterus.

There are other explanations, however. In the UK, pagan people may believe the energies of the Earth influence conception, and that the locus of the land at conception is important. In contrast, amongst both rural and urban Indian and African populations, there is consensus about the critical role of ancestors in ensuring conception occurs. Examples given below from the ethnographic literature illustrate the multiple theories of pregnancy causation.

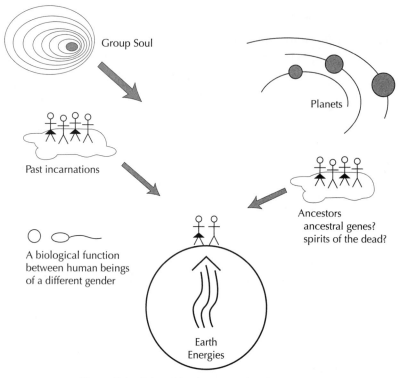

Figure 5.1. Cultural Explanations for Conception

What is involved in conception?

The anthropologist Reichel-Dolmatoff (1997) has explained that the Tukano in the Amazon rainforest believed the sun was the main energy in the universe, rather than any 'divinity', and it was linked with the life force and with sperm. The Tukano agreed that a woman's uterus was like a cooking pot, potentially fertile, and when a child was born, it was considered to be a container for solar energy.

Likewise in Africa, the Dinka of Sudan believed conception occurred only with divinity, or with some kind of divine presence. According to the anthropologist Lienhardt (1990, p.39), the population explained it was 'divinity' which created a child inside a woman's belly and had 'a creative function in the formation of every human being'. One might think divine intervention was present in 2013 when a clothing factory collapsed in Dakar, Bangladesh: a woman gave birth to a live baby boy while underneath the rubble, which killed more than 1000 people.

Proscriptions during pregnancy

In Malaysia, a husband had to refrain from hunting during his wife's pregnancy, or the foetus of his unborn child would be wounded in the same way as he wounded the hunted animal. During labour, all doors and windows should be kept open to ensure an easy birth (Hurlbut 1992). In neighbouring Indonesia, among the Laboya, similar taboos controlled the husband's hunting activities during a woman's pregnancy (Geirnaert-Martin 1992).

In addition, for populations from countries like India and among the diaspora from South Asia, the alignment of the planets was very important regarding marriage, conception and the future life of the child and adult. In some countries, beliefs included the role of past incarnations as influences on the fertility of either prospective parent. For example, in cases where populations held reincarnation beliefs, it was important that a person had behaved carefully and morally in a previous life: both one's own and one's ancestors, as otherwise this might influence an unborn child.

Role of ancestors in conception

The possibility that conception occurred by the will of an ancestral soul resulted in various Indian cultures' concern with having a 'good' or untroubled death, so that ancestors could reincarnate as a new baby and not remain in limbo like ghosts (Parry 1994, Obeyesekere 1981 and Fuller 1992). However, someone who died a bad death could get stuck in a liminal state as a ghost and be blocked from being reborn.

Ancestral relationships affected the health and wellbeing of people in different ways. In countries like India and Sri Lanka, where people believed conception occurred by the will of an ancestral soul, this resulted in a concern by various cultures with having a 'good' death so that the ancestors could reincarnate and not remain in limbo like ghosts. In Asia, people believed malevolent spirits took possession of the living and controlled their minds and bodies.

The idea that spirits existed in some kind of non-physical dimension and overshadowed human beings was found in many societies which had a belief in existence after death. In the west, if a discarnate being appears to the recently bereaved as a hallucination or apparition, this may be considered delusional or a case of 'complicated grief', whereas in other societies it might be a welcome vision.

These beliefs were found closer to home when the French ethnographer, Capdecomme (1998), conducted a research project in a village in Wales in the 1990s where the psychics and mediums were mostly women. They claimed that ghosts who came to trouble the living were those who had been unhappy alive, or who had experienced a brutal or sudden death, or who had not been appropriately prayed over. People considered it was proof that not only an individual's personality survived but also the relationships that they had had. Good ghosts came back with messages, with affection and tranquillity. When they spoke, they talked about the future. They helped people understand human nature. Bad ghosts created mental health problems.

In northern Alberta in Canada, the Dene Tha indigenous people held similar beliefs. They drove cars and trucks, had televisions and abided by the Roman Catholic faith. However, they said although sexual intercourse was necessary for procreation, it was not sufficient: it occurred through the souls of their ancestors who wanted to be reborn. Their underlying belief was that a foetus was always the result of the death and regeneration of an ancestor.

Perhaps medical and healthcare providers in the UK and abroad might find it useful to be aware of a different focus of beliefs in other cultures. People believed ancestors could influence conception both through genes and through spirits of the dead who could benevolently support a conception: it was the ancestors who recycled in order to create a new-born. However, consensus also suggested that earthbound ancestors or ghosts could cause mischief to people if they had not moved off the Earth's plane.

Further afield, to the north-east of Australia are the Trobriand Islands of New Guinea. Malinowski the anthropologist who visited said Trobriand islanders in the early twentieth century claimed they were 'so mixed up with beliefs about the incarnations of spiritual beings' that he had to address biological and spiritual ideas together (1929, p.145). Beliefs about birth and death were intertwined. Islanders believed ancestral spirits were the real cause of conception and childbirth. In this book, beliefs about death and beyond are discussed in more detail in Chapters 8 and 9.

Babies, human identity and soul

In the UK, spiritualist practitioners consider that individuals descend into a woman's womb from a group soul. Others believe that the soul is continuous and simply inhabits a body during its time on earth – once the body dies, the soul returns to the group of origin. Some Chinese people believe that the spirit of the child is already wandering around before birth, so an unborn child is treated as if it is already there. There are many other proscriptions regarding food and actions for the traditional Chinese mother-to-be.

Cultural beliefs about a new-born baby

Once a baby has been born, there are a number of non-physical elements which make up a human being: these include the body, self, soul, spirit, breath and life force. Beliefs about the nature of elements making up a new-born baby influence the kind of health-seeking strategies that the population undertake in times of illness.

Common consensus means that populations in different countries hold different assumptions about the components which make up a new-born. As well as biological aspects, the Sabarl of Papua New Guinea believed that *hinona* (the essence of life, vital substance) made up the body and the breath (Battaglia 1990). Among Malay peoples, components of a new-born include: the soul (*ruh*), the breath of life (*nyawa*) and the spirit of life (*semangat*) (Laderman 1982). People believed the life force could leave the body and this was especially risky in a new-born.

In Thailand, the anthropologist Ruth Inge Heinze observed that once a baby was born, ceremonies took place to ensure it stayed on earth. The *tham khwan* ceremony used cotton thread to tie the life force or soul into a new-born (Heinze 1982). A thread was tied to ensure the baby returned in case they wandered to other realms during sleep. The *khwan* was 'the essence of life' and it entered a woman's womb at conception. The life force was an invisible component of a person. As a child grew, its *khwan* grew too and became more attached to its physical body. It was indestructible but could leave the body during sleep and roam around for short periods, similar to the practice of lucid dreaming or shamanic journeying.

A child was considered to be both an individual bound by skin and a person that had a permeable body. A new-born consisted of a body, breath and a soul and its identity was not fixed at the skin. A new-born's flesh was considered to be permeable and potentially its body was susceptible to the attention of 'spirit beings'. Prophylactic measures were used by some peoples against supernatural attack during childbirth in Borneo. When I was in Sudan, I also saw relatives place a metal knife blade under the place where the new mother and baby slept to avert the evil eye.

Children's reincarnation memories

In many societies, a being's identity is rooted within the local cosmology even before conception. Among the Trobriand islanders, the deceased are part of the cycle of the living: it is their 'souls' which reincarnate into a foetus. In addition, among the Dene Tha in Canada, a young child may have recollections of the individual he or she once was in previous life. They may have birthmarks relating to a previous incarnation and this information becomes part of the child's sense of identity. The Druze in Palestine and Israel also hold reincarnation beliefs.

The psychiatrist Ian Stevenson was head of department at the University of Virginia's school of medicine, Charlottesville. He was famous for investigating reports of children who claimed to remember a past life and the events that occurred during a previous life. He published over 2,500 case studies and claimed memories normally occurred in children between three and seven years of age and then fade.

He believed the evidence most suggestive of reincarnation was the existence of birthmarks and deformities on children, particularly when they occurred at the location of fatal wounds (in the person who had died). The majority of cases investigated appeared to involve those who met a violent or untimely death. About 35% of children who claimed to remember previous lives had birthmarks and/or birth defects, which they attributed to wounds on the person whose life they remembered. This topic is addressed again in Chapter 9 on beliefs about survival beyond death.

Midwifery of the deceased and the new-born

Weiner (1976) was an anthropologist who visited Papua New Guinea 50 years after Malinowski. She noticed women on the islands were responsible for the funerary rites of the dead since these involved the birth of a new ancestor. In Papua New Guinea, new mothers and recently widowed women also wore the same dress: one ushered in a new birth, the other a new ancestor.

Similarly in Indonesia, Laboya pregnant women were considered to be containers of the ancestral breath and spirit (*mawo* and *dewa*) and as such they were believed to be temporarily in touch with the 'realm of the dead'. In these countries, common consensus maintained that the cycle of death and birth was intricately linked together. When new migrants arrive in Western countries, we may need to consider their range of beliefs when they seek healthcare services.

MIDWIFERY

The attitudes to and consensus about midwifery have changed over the centuries and I have included this to illustrate the cultural U-turns which have occurred in the profession. After the Middle Ages, women were increasingly excluded from attending births: midwifery became linked to superstition and witchcraft. During the eighteenth century, there was a struggle for control of childbirth between midwives and the emerging, male-dominated medical profession. Before the 1800s, women in labour were traditionally attended by female relatives or friends, with untrained female midwives or traditional birth attendants.

Midwifery had its origins in social welfare and public health. Social reformers, suffragettes and some medical practitioners lobbied for the first Midwifery Act in 1902. It did not come from a specialist branch of nursing. Many female midwives were skilled at manual delivery and had great practical knowledge about birth and birthing. They did not usually use instruments. The use of obstetric forceps and caesarean section by male physicians and surgeons allowed them to deliver babies when, otherwise, the mother and/or baby would have died.

The Midwives Act 1902 forced women to choose between legal, registered midwifery of birth or midwifery of the dead. Meanwhile, in Africa, traditional birth attendants (TBA) were not necessarily trained but were women who knew about the need for quality care of mother and child. These days TBAs are trained in obstetrics to support their communities. 'So God dealt well with the midwives; and the people multiplied and became very strong' (Exodus 1.20, NRSV).

The nineteenth century onwards saw a progressive medicalization and male dominance of pregnancy and childbirth. At this time, a pregnant woman came to be seen as a 'patient'. Pregnancy was increasingly portrayed as pathological and needing close medical surveillance. During the mid-twentieth century, there was a trend towards routine anaesthesia, with increasing rates of instrument delivery and caesarean section.

In the UK, there was a change in consensus about the 'best' place for births to take place. For example, in 1927 only 15% of babies were born in hospitals or other institutions, but by 1959, a third of births occurred at home or in nursing homes. However, by 1985, consensus meant that 99% of births were in NHS hospitals. Care seemed to become about 'processing' women through birth without incident. For a while, treatment focused on producing a 'perfect' baby and working with a mother's physiology for this purpose.

Despite campaigning by the home birth movement, by 2011 only 2.5% of all births were at home. The South West of England had the highest percentage of women giving birth at home in 2011 (3.5%), while the North East had the lowest (1.0%). The current underlying assumption is that home births are not as safe as hospital births.

SUMMARY

In this chapter, I have looked at the concept of personhood and self. I have also presented ancient wisdoms from some societies to depict what they believed made up a human being from a spiritual perspective. I have explored a variety of beliefs about what a human being consists of, the different understandings of being born free and the soul, life force and the self. There was the first mention of the notion that the self can wander during sleep – this is mentioned in later chapters when addressing the centre of perception as being beyond the body, like in a shamanic journey.

I have also considered the profound relationship between birth and death and ancestral beings, which so many people adhere to. This belief influenced how people thought babies were made. I have illustrated a variety of influences on conception which goes beyond the biological egg and sperm explanation.

Beliefs from the ethnographic literature were introduced about reincarnation memories and I noted that midwifery used to be a service of the dead, where ancestors resulted in new conceptions and subsequent births. I have noted the changes in attitude that occurred around western midwifery.

This chapter has presented a range of cultural explanations for conception and also cultural understandings of the non-physical elements of a human body. There was a brief review of eighteenth- and nineteenth-century midwifery. The ways in which social attitudes and the common consensus have changed in terms of birth, sex outside of marriage and adoption are covered in Chapter 7.

6

WOMEN'S BODIES AND HUMAN BEHAVIOUR

In this chapter, I explore the status and value of women and consider ways in which these may change and be culturally different in some communities. I look at a variety of models of 'the family' and present beliefs about the ideal kind of human behaviour and actual human behaviour, which may be quite different.

There are various factors women experience which influence their wellbeing. These include arranged and forced marriage, the concepts of honour and shame, strategies for attack, circumcision (female genital mutilation (FGM) or cutting), the practice of rape and the occurrence of spirit possession.

Some of these things we may be familiar with and others have found their way into popular newspapers. There are distressing things mentioned here in this section on women which may also happen to men. I will cover things which some people in some societies may consider to be outrageously wrong, whereas those people in those places where they are done consider them to be normal.

In order to deepen our understanding of the ways consensus changes over time, I will explore the value of women, their bodies and a few life events. The aim is to raise awareness of cultural beliefs which influence access to healthcare. It is also to emphasize that cultural U-turns occur over time and geographical location. Events occur that trigger U-turns and one I will mention is the rape and death of a young woman in India.

WOMEN, MARRIAGE AND FAMILIES
A normal family model

Let us look at different types of family arrangements that exist in the west. These include: the nuclear family, where both parents and children live together as a unit; the single parent family, where children are brought up living with only one parent; extended families where children, parents and other family members live together as a unit or nearby; the reconstituted family, where two sets of children become one family when their divorced parents marry each other; and, cohabiting parents where parents live together but have not married.

In earlier times, travellers to India used to make assumptions about what was right and normal. For example, when early psychologists travelled from the UK to India in the 1950s, they assumed Indian families did not take good care of their children, as they were often left with extended family members. The consensus assumption was that the observer's model of the nuclear family was the 'correct' one, and other models were of less value or wrong. Of course, we don't tend to make these kinds of assumptions today, but we might make them in other areas of people's lives with which we are less familiar.

During a mental health research project I carried out with the Somali community (Tobert 2010b), data showed the word 'family' included a person's extended family, and not just the nuclear family. When asked who was a brother, people included a male person of the same religion or the same country. Only 30% considered a woman of the same clan to be a sister.

A question of honour

Honour killing is the murder of a woman accused of bringing shame upon her family. In the UK, murders sometimes take place after a family reacts violently to their son or daughter taking on western culture. It may be carried out by the father and brothers of the woman. Killings are often disguised as suicides, a fire or an accident. Police believe there may be as many as 12 honour killings in the UK every year. They may occur within Asian or Near and Middle Eastern families when a person is believed to have 'dishonoured' their loved ones.

Honour attacks using acid sometimes occur in countries from the Near East and Asia (Afghanistan, Iran, Pakistan and India) with the aim of disfiguring another's face (Bandyopadhyay *et al.* 2003). They also happen at times in parts of Africa and South Asia. Incidents occur with abusers claiming they are punishing women for 'sullying family honour' by 'indecent' behaviour, like being improperly veiled. This practice is not supported by either political or religious leaders (Taylor 2000).

A BBC report in 2011 informed us that honour attacks were punishments, usually but not always on women, for acts deemed to have brought shame on their nuclear or extended family. In 2010, 39 UK police forces recorded 2,823 'honour' attacks. However, 12 forces were unable or unwilling to provide data as communities were reluctant to talk about the crime and may even deny the existence of honour attacks.

Eight police forces each recorded more than 100 honour-based attacks: the Metropolitan Police (495), Bedfordshire (117), West Midlands (378), West Yorkshire (350), Lancashire (227), Greater Manchester (189), Cleveland (153) and Suffolk (118). These attacks included acid, abduction, mutilation, beating and, in some cases, murder. In the UK there were over 100 acid attacks in 2014.

In the UK, the domestic violence training for officers of the Metropolitan Police included issues of honour-based violence and forced marriages: 32 London boroughs had a community safety unit, with over 560 specially trained officers. They said that '[w]e know that like other hate crimes, honour-based violence is underreported, and [we] remain very concerned about this' (BBC n.d.).

One Home Office spokesman stated:

> 'We are determined to end honour violence and recognize the need for greater consistency on the ground to stop this indefensible practice. Our action plan to end violence against women and girls sets out our approach to raise awareness, enhance training for police and prosecutors and better support victims.' (BBC 2011)

Attempts have been made to end the silence surrounding honour attacks. A charity, Karma Nirvana, was set up in Derby after one woman's sister killed herself to escape marriage. Its helpline opened in April 2008 and received 4,000 calls during the first year of its existence. It takes 300 calls a month from people under the threat of honour-based violence, often linked to forced marriage. When women escape forced marriage in the UK, they live with the fear and rejection of their families, communities and friends. The same applies to gay men, who may be forced into marriage.

Arranged and forced marriage

In 1948, the United Nations set out the Universal Declaration of Human Rights which stated that 'marriage shall be entered into only with the free and full consent of the intending spouses'. In the UK, the Foreign Office (2013) set out clear guidelines on the differences between arranged and forced marriages. With an arranged marriage, a person has a choice as to whether to accept the arrangement or not.

This tradition of arranged marriages has operated successfully within many communities and countries for a very long time. However, with a forced marriage, a man or a woman is coerced into marrying someone against their will. They may be physically threatened or emotionally blackmailed. It is an abuse of human rights and is not justified on any religious or cultural basis.

In the UK, the Forced Marriage Unit was a joint initiative developed with the Home Office. In 2012, that office gave advice or support to 1485 cases: 82% were female and 18% were male.

CIRCUMCISION
Female circumcision

The Foundation for Women's Health estimated that nearly 66,000 women who had undergone FGM were living in England and Wales. Over 20,000 girls under five were at risk of FGM or may have been subjected to one of the different types. The foundation suggested that the procedure violated a girl's right to good health and protection from the pre-meditated infliction of grievous genital harm. The practice occurs in 28 countries, to women of various religion and ethnicities, including Muslims and Christians.

In 2008, when I ran a discussion group with African and Asian women in the London borough of Harrow, there were different perspectives: African Muslim and Christian women considered female circumcision to be a normal practice, whereas Asian Muslim women had not heard of the practice. There was a general awareness that girls were taken out of school to travel back to their country of origin to have the procedure. In that group there was no consensus: some

African women thought the practice did no harm, whilst Asian women were shocked by it.

In 1997, the World Health Organization (WHO 2016) defined female circumcision as 'all procedures involving partial or total removal of the external female genitalia or other injury to the female genital organs whether for cultural or non-therapeutic reasons'. The procedure affected 150 million women worldwide.

Among peoples in those countries, it was a normal cultural practice. However, another term in current use for female circumcision is FGM, which suggests that although the practice of the procedure is widespread, it is not universally condoned. In the UK, one organization among many set up to combat the practice is Afruca (Africans Unite against Child Abuse).[1]

Living in the UK, around 20,000 girls are thought to be at risk of female circumcision and a story about FGM featured on prime-time television for the first time on a Saturday evening drama, *Casualty*. The storyline was about a girl who had undergone the procedure and was trying to protect her younger sister from the same fate. The younger sister was threatened with being forced to travel abroad to her extended family for the cutting.

In 1985, the UK government passed the Female Circumcision Prohibition Act which made it illegal for anyone to carry out the practice within the United Kingdom. However, although it was illegal for any resident of the UK to perform FGM within or outside the UK, this didn't mean to say it did not happen. The punishment for violating the revised 2003 Act carried 14 years imprisonment, a fine or both. Two men were convicted in London for carrying out the procedure.

In some communities, FGM was mistakenly believed to be a religious requirement and an obligation. In others, there was social acceptance whereby people believed uncircumcised girls and women were unclean, promiscuous and unmarriageable. A majority of Africans who used the procedure were either Christians or Muslims, yet neither the Bible nor the Koran supported the practice.

The Bible is silent on FGM. The command from God to have Abraham remove the foreskins of his sons through circumcision is very clear in Genesis, but it is important to note that nowhere in

---

1   www.afruca.org

the Bible is it mentioned that any female children or grown women should be circumcised. With regard to the Quran, Sheikh Mohammed Sayyid Tantawi categorically stated: 'FGM has neither been mentioned in Quran nor Sunnah'.[2] This was reaffirmed by a top official cleric and Grand Mufti of Egypt, Sheikh Ali Gomma. He said 'Prophet Mohammed didn't circumcise his four daughters'. In addition, Sheikh Yousif Algaradawi avowed that 'FGM is not an Islamic requirement'.

Female circumcision is an example of what has been normal in some places, but it is against the law in the UK. The cultural U-turn occurred recently in the UK with raised awareness about the practice thanks to African celebrities.

Rape

Rape is the unlawful compelling of a person through physical force or the threat of violence to submit to an act of sexual intercourse. Sexual violence without consent may be perpetrated by a complete stranger or by someone known and trusted. Rape occurs to men as well as women, but we will address the latter here.

In 2012, an incident of gang rape which occurred on a bus in India and resulted in the death of the female victim was significant. This was because the aftermath of the act appeared to result in a shift in societal awareness from common consensus on or silence about or acceptance of the status quo, changing to action in thought and deed throughout India.

TRIGGERS FOR THE CULTURAL U-TURN AGAINST RAPE IN INDIA

After a woman's death in December 2012, thousands of mourning Indians lit candles, held prayer meetings to express grief and marched through cities and towns, including New Delhi, Mumbai, Bangalore and Kolkata. Scuffles broke out in central Delhi between police and protesters who said their government was doing too little to protect women. The protests spread across India and raised questions about lax attitudes by the police to sexual crimes.

---

2   http://forwarduk.org.uk/female-genital-mutilation-not-islamic-say-top-egyptian-clerics

As a result of the suffering and death of this anonymous young woman, people in India gathered to say no to rape, but observers noted contradictions as people took a reflective look at social mores. As the Al Jazeera reporter Dinesh Sharma noted: 'Indians pray to goddesses in temples, but abuse women in [the] domestic sphere. They elect women to powerful political offices, yet mistreat girls in public.'[3]

There was a claim that gender bias prevented women from reporting crimes of rape: 'This bias, cloaked under the notion of family or community "honour", effectively serves to silence the voices of many women survivors of violence.'[4] Previously in India, rapes were dramatically under-reported, and of the ones reported, the police recorded few and verified fewer still. In addition, the crime of rape tended to blame and shame victims, minimizing the offence and letting perpetrators off the hook.

The crime galvanized people to demand greater protection for women from sexual violence. The students of Jawaharlal Nehru University in South Delhi marched silently to the bus stop where the bus in question was boarded. The Chief Minister of West Bengal pledged 65 all-female police stations to deal with crimes against women. Ranjana Kumari (2012), Director of the Centre for Social Research in New Delhi, noted:

> This is an unprecedented response to this rape case not only because of its sheer brutality that moved them beyond imagination but also because we have so many rape cases reported over the years and our justice system is really very slow and conviction rates are very, very low...rape cases are...increasing because there is no fear of law at the moment and people want all this to change.

The funeral of the student who died was a time for deep reflection in India. Her ashes were scattered over the River Ganges. Hundreds lined the banks of the sacred river to pay their respects with the victim's family. The funeral procession took three hours to cover five miles because so many participated.

Kavita Krishnan, the secretary of the All India Progressive Women's Association (AIPWA) said it was time 'to think about women's position in society and the various ways in which [they face] inequality and

---

3   www.aljazeera.com/indepth/opinion/2012/12/201212319356987371.html
4   www.aljazeera.com/indepth/opinion/2012/12/2012122184411816140.html

injustice' (Nandi and Ghosal 2012). There was a further claim that Indian women were participating in genocide against female foetuses because their culture sanctioned it.

Problems of being female in India

During the twentieth century, there were certain problems associated with 'being female' in India. The population was skewed: families had strong preferences for sons over daughters and this led to sex-selective abortions. Female foetuses were aborted and baby girls were killed after birth. Furthermore, over two million women went missing in any given year: 12% disappeared at birth; 25% died in childhood; 18% died at reproductive age and 45% died at older ages. Each year, more than 100,000 women were killed in accidents by fire (Biswas 2012).

The economists Anderson and Ray have suggested that deep-rooted changes in social attitudes are needed to make India's women more accepted and secure and to address widespread misogyny. Selectively aborting a female foetus does occur in the UK, and reporters claim the global practice has led to a shortfall of millions of girls throughout the world (ibid).

A flurry of reporters commented on the situation:

"When I look at the thousands of protesters on the streets demanding a firm law, more policing and justice for the rape victim, my thoughts go to a place where rape is born, in our very homes...I look around to see a million women silently living each day the horrific incident that happened to them, not by a stranger but by a loved one: an uncle, a husband maybe a grandfather or a father. But they live in silence because that is what they were taught." This journalist reported that mothers should say: "we will not tell our daughters to shut up and live with it".[5]

Changes are happening in India and cultural U-turns are occurring within the courts of justice. In New Delhi, a court recently ruled that a woman can be the legal head of a family, which in the past was a position reserved for men. As legal head, a woman occupies a senior position and has control over property and prayer rituals.

---

5 http://timesofindia.indiatimes.com/home/The-rapes-that-we-dont-talk-about/articleshow/17805523.cms

UK, G8 meeting on rape and war

To what extent are images from India and the changes in social awareness transferable to the UK? There was a meeting in April 2013 about the topic of rape and war. The G8 Foreign Ministers met in London. The actress Angelina Jolie attended the meeting, joining Foreign Secretary William Hague (2013) to raise awareness about sexual violence in military conflicts. She focused on wartime rape: 'it is encouraging to see men in leadership positions speaking out against rape. Rape is not a women's issue, or a humanitarian issue, it is a global issue.' Millions of pounds were given by G8 ministers to create changes in attitudes about rape and war.[6]

SUMMARY

The chapter has looked at several models of the family and the assumptions made in the past about what was a 'normal' family. I have presented beliefs about the ideal kind of human behaviour, and actual human behaviour, which is rather different. I have discussed topics such as the differences between arranged and forced marriage, honour attacks, the concept of shame and rape and I have noted different attitudes towards FGM.

I have explored the status and value of women and the ways these were culturally different. Practices like female circumcision occurred not only in Central Africa, but also elsewhere in the world, where they were carried out by Christian and Muslim families. Female infanticide was regarded as normal by some people and practised in certain parts of the world.

There is clearly a need to be able to communicate during a medical or healthcare consultation, so that each person is heard and acknowledged, without passing judgment on a cultural practice that does not fit one's own religious or social background. The practice of Open Dialogue, which is gaining favour, appears to be a suitable communication strategy if it considers cultural beliefs alongside mindfulness, dialogue and compassion.

---

6   www.gov.uk/government/news/g8-declaration-on-preventing-sexual-violence-in-conflict

7

CULTURAL U-TURNS AND CHANGING RESPONSES TO CONSENSUS

In this chapter, I discuss how the things I have mentioned so far in this book have changed over time. I present a series of U-turns that societies have taken. I summarize our changing consensus on various topics, and in particular I start to ask how the diagnosis and treatment of mental illness have changed over time. I explore ways in which our social consensus has changed since the ancient incarceration of people with symptoms and our understanding of the triggers of distress.

Why am I exploring the nature of changing common consensus and health? I began this book because I wanted to explore the extent to which change happened. I wanted to see how social, religious and community leaders achieved consensus and then radically changed their minds about it over time. People who questioned the agreed norm of polite society could be deemed mentally deficient.

It was obvious to me that there appeared to have been huge shifts in public understanding and awareness about human activities and behaviour and profound policy changes at a state level regarding human health.

I chose to gather evidence to illustrate cultural U-turns in order to illustrate that radical change has occurred in the past. I suggest that change is normal. I wanted to put forward the proposition that deep change is possible again in the future, particularly in the field of spiritual approaches to health and mental wellbeing. I address these issues in later chapters.

In this section I explore changing social attitudes and the reframing of common consensus on the following topics: birth, sex outside of marriage, illegitimacy, adoption and mental health diagnoses. Finally, I illustrate historical assumptions about children born out of wedlock and the criminal records given in the past to those who practised homosexual activities. We have changed our attitudes.

CHANGES IN CONSENSUS AROUND CHILDREN
Fast medical U-turn

In 2014, one couple sparked an international police hunt when they took their sick son with a brain tumour from a hospital in Southampton. The boy's parents wanted to take him abroad for proton beam therapy, which had fewer side effects than radiotherapy. The parents were later arrested and imprisoned for 24 hours. However, the High Court gave permission for the boy to be treated.

Within 18 months of the police hunt, the *Lancet* had published an article saying that photon beam therapy was effective with few side effects for children in his condition (Yock *et al.* 2016). In this case, the researchers were reviewing the topic before it had reached the mainstream medical press. It looked like a very fast medical U-turn.

Forced adoption (UK)

In the western world, our beliefs about conception and birth have changed over the past few decades. In the 1950s and 60s, we maintained one set of beliefs about pregnancy and sex outside of marriage, which decades later has changed radically. We (society) used to believe that any woman who had sex outside of marriage was mentally deficient (Pollack 2013, Paton 2012), and if her baby was conceived out of wedlock, then that baby was also born mentally deficient, or did not deserve a Christian burial (Crandell 2014).

In the past, adoptions took place due to social pressures on women who had children outside marriage. Jean Robertson-Molloy was from the Movement for an Adoption Apology (MAA) campaign (Roberts 2013). This was started in 2010 to demand a cross-party parliamentary apology for past adoption practices.

The group wanted governments to recognize suffering caused by forced adoptions during the 1950s, 1960s and 1970s and to acknowledge the unacceptable adoption and care practices of the past towards single mothers. They were not offered information about welfare services, housing and financial help, though this was available at the time. Furthermore, they had not questioned whether those women putting their children up for adoption had given their informed consent.

Manchester MP John Leech joined the campaigning and submitted a motion for debate in the House of Commons, asking for a government apology for unmarried mothers. The BBC transmitted a radio programme entitled *The Crying Shame* by presenter Phil Frampton. He had visited the unmarried mothers' home in St Agnes, Cornwall, where he was born in 1953.

Frampton said: 'my mother was a Birmingham teacher. Not being married she bore me in secret to avoid bringing shame.' 'Mothers were systematically humiliated, forced to watch from a locked room as the adopters drove their baby away.' Through common consensus, this was considered normal: institutions carrying out these acts were publicly funded through the Church of England and local authorities. At the time, babies of 'mixed-race' parentage like Phil Frampton were considered to have a physical defect.

Martin Narey, a former CEO at Barnardo's, claimed children from ethnic minorities were over-represented amongst those seeking adoption. He said the law was very clear: a child should not stay in care for an undue length of time while waiting for adoptive parents of the same ethnicity. 'But the reality is that African, Asian and mixed race children wait three times longer than white children.'[1]

It seems consensus has changed considerably during our lifetimes. There are behaviours, which local authorities, governments and religious institutions assumed were appropriate some decades ago, whereas they now consider that the consensus agreement at that time was seriously flawed. Cultural U-turns became normal practice.

Forced adoption (Australia)

The attitudes towards sex outside of wedlock also existed in Australia. In spring 2013, former Prime Minister Julia Gillard issued an apology to people affected by their forced adoption policy between the 1950s

---

1   www.bbc.co.uk/news/education-12258379

and 1970s. At that time, tens of thousands of babies of unmarried, mostly teenage mothers were taken by the state and given to childless married couples.

A Senate inquiry report was published based on submissions from hundreds of women. Many said they had given up their children because of the stigma attached to unmarried motherhood at the time. Some said they were drugged, while others said their signatures were forged.

Today, many women say they were coerced into signing away their children. Mothers had been denied knowledge of their rights: they could not provide informed consent. Many women were forced to live in maternity homes until their delivery. Once in hospital, some described being tied to the bed.

At Parliament House, Canberra the former Prime Minister Gillard said:

> Today, this Parliament, on behalf of the Australian people, takes responsibility and apologizes for the policies and practices that forced the separation of mothers from their babies which created a lifelong legacy of pain and suffering. We deplore the shameful practices that denied you, the mothers, your fundamental rights and responsibilities to love and care for your children.
>
> You were given false assurances: you were forced to endure the coercion and brutality of practices that were unethical, dishonest and in many cases illegal.
>
> By saying sorry, we can correct the historical record. We can declare that these mothers did nothing wrong, that you loved your children and you always will.[2]

One mother who had her child sent for adoption explained her perspective: 'The trauma of enforced separation from my first-born child has resulted in lifelong psychological distress to both me and my daughter.' 'I gave birth to my first child, a girl, in 1964. She was collected from hospital by her adoptive parents after ten days.'[3]

---

2   www.ag.gov.au/About/ForcedAdoptionsApology/Pages/default.aspx; www.dss.gov.
     au/our-responsibilities/families-and-children/programs-services/forced-adoption-
     practices; www.npr.org/sections/thetwo-way/2013/03/20/174890534/australian-
     prime-minister-apologizes-for-forced-adoption-policy
3   https://open.abc.net.au/explore/29631

In 1982, a child psychiatrist said he was surprised how many of his patients were told their child would be better off – this had a profoundly negative effect on a mother and her subsequent children.

The stolen generation

In Australia during the twentieth century, common consensus agreed on what are now regarded as racist issues concerning Aboriginal children and the 'stolen generation' for which there is deep regret today. Between 1910 and 1970, the Australian government took 100,000 Aboriginal children, many of them under five years old, away from their homes (Manne 2001). They were taken away from their families because the government did not believe in the future of the Aborigines. They thought it would be better to bring them up with white families.

In 1995, an investigation was opened to bring more truth to the topic, but at that time the government did not apologize to victims. The National Inquiry into the Separation of Aboriginal and Torres Strait Islander Children from their Families was entitled 'Bringing Them Home' (Lenzerini 2009). Prime Minister Kevin Rudd was the first Australian politician to make a formal apology to the Aborigines in 2008. There was the example of Bruce Trevorrow who was taken in 1957 and sent to a white foster family. Later in life he suffered from depression and turned to alcohol. In 1998, he went to court and won approximately half a million dollars from the Australian government as a form of compensation.

The movement in Australia to remove Aboriginal children from their parents was appropriate according to peer agreement and the common consensus at the time. The same thing happened during the nineteenth and twentieth centuries to indigenous Native American children, who were systematically removed from their mothers and adopted by white families in an attempt to integrate them into settler ways. This occurred until the 1978 Indian Child Welfare Act.

Canada also practised cultural genocide for over a century, forcing around 150,000 indigenous children into Indian residential schools run by the Church (TRC). They wanted the children to live 'like whites' and as children were taken from their parents and their siblings, there were many suicides (25% of students).

One of the confessions of the Presbyterian Church in 1994 seems illustrative of a change of direction:

> In our cultural arrogance we have been blind to the ways in which our own understanding of the Gospel has been culturally conditioned, and because of our insensitivity to Aboriginal cultures, we have demanded more of the Aboriginal people than the Gospel requires, and have thus misrepresented Jesus Christ who loves all peoples with compassionate, suffering love that all may come to God through him. For the Church's presumption we ask forgiveness. (Truth and Reconciliation Commission of Canada 2015, p.282)

Several decades later, what looked like a normal consensual twentieth-century practice seemed by twenty-first century social mores to be inhumane, racist, hugely damaging and socially inappropriate. These things required far-reaching cultural U-turns from the Church and government alike.

The mental health of children born out of wedlock

Common consensus changes over time and space: our attitude towards sex outside of marriage and the deficiencies of babies born out of wedlock has changed. In the past, governments and religious institutions agreed to take a set of actions which later – starting from 2013 – they apologized for. These included forced adoptions, children 'stolen' for re-schooling and the fact that some mothers were considered 'defective' and placed within the mental health system. This was a time when a child of mixed race was considered a defect and the concepts of shame and humiliation were ubiquitous. This occurred in the twentieth century. To what extent have we changed?

Unmarried mothers, unmarried fathers and their children born outside marriage were considered deviants. All were called 'illegitimate' and were considered legally and socially inferior to legitimate families headed by married couples. In the nineteenth and early twentieth centuries, there was a widespread belief that children born out of wedlock posed significant social and public health problems.

Illegitimacy was considered a major factor in mental deficiency, disease and anti-social behaviour. The assumption was that illegitimate pregnancies were by-products of insanity and other mental defects. In the 1970s, unmarried mothers were discovered in mental asylums, having been incarcerated for decades. In Ireland, the offspring of unmarried mothers were also believed to be mentally ill due to the nature of their conception. What other aspects of our life and health have changed over time or among different cultures?

MENTAL HEALTH AND BEING GAY: CULTURAL U-TURNS

Over the years, some societies have changed their minds about homosexuality. The British mathematician Dr Alan Turing had played a key role in breaking the German Enigma code, and this considerably shortened the Second World War. In 1952, he was convicted for gross indecency and this meant he could not obtain security clearance to continue working at GCHQ (Government Communications Headquarters), a government intelligence agency. He then lost his job. He was chemically castrated following his conviction for the crime of gross indecency: sexual activity with a man. His work was said to be pivotal to the development of modern computing. In 1954, he committed suicide.

In December 2013, Turing was granted a posthumous royal pardon by the Queen under the Royal Prerogative of Mercy (Grayling 2013). Gay rights campaigners have suggested that there are more than 50,000 less famous men who also received criminal convictions for homosexual relationships in the twentieth century. Their cases also need to be considered.

In 2012, a seventy-three-year old UK pensioner, John Crawford, fought to clear a criminal record he received in the 1950s for being in a consensual gay relationship. He applied to have the conviction annulled and had discovered his criminal record on applying for voluntary work: 'I looked back over my life and realized that all the work I'd lost over the years was due to this criminal record.' 'I came into this world without a criminal record and I don't want to die with a criminal record.' [4] There are around 16,000 people in the UK with a sexual offences record, even though their actions are now deemed legal.

The cultural U-turn occurred in 1967 when the offences were decriminalized but the previous convictions remained. In 2012, the

---

4   www.bbc.co.uk/news/uk-england-london-20522465

Protection of Freedoms Act gained Royal Assent and changed the law so historical convictions for decriminalized consensual sex offences did not appear on criminal record checks. However, those affected still needed to apply to the Home Secretary for a former conviction to be annulled.

The problems of being gay and Asian or Muslim or African still remain in certain geographical locations. For example, there may be additional pressure on Muslim men: homosexuality is forbidden in many Muslim countries, as is suicide. The assumption is that 'there is no such thing as a gay Muslim'. The subject of being a religious, practising Muslim and gay is taboo. Men may be forced into marriages to protect their family's reputation. A cycle of events may occur: they may lie to their wives, flee their marriages, become homeless or face rejection by their family and peers. All these factors may keep Muslim gay men isolated. However, individual imams or priests may help men to reconcile themselves with their faith.

This means that while in some parts of the world consensus has changed with regard to homosexual practice, in other societies, it is still taboo. In the same geographical place, at the same time, among people of different cultural origins, consensus is not consistent. The Anglican Church was divided over homosexuality during its talks with 38 Church leaders in Canterbury (Sherwood 2016). However, Pope Frances said: 'If someone is gay and he searches for the Lord and has good will, who am I to judge? We shouldn't marginalize people for this. They must be integrated into society.'

CHANGING EXPLANATORY MODELS FOR MENTAL DISTRESS

In the previous section, I illustrated some cultural U-terns which have taken place. However, cultural consensus on interpretations of mental distress may be contemporaneous at the same place or at different places. Different cultures residing in the same geographic location may possess a wide range of cultural explanatory models for mental distress.

In addition, people belonging to the same 'culture' may possess quite different opinions about interpreting symptoms.

Consensus on incarceration and mental health

In order to begin to explore the ways in which the consensus on mental health has changed over the last decade, I will start with an introduction to the Testimony Project. This was an archive of 50 interviews conducted between 1999 and 2000 which were stored at the British Library.

In 2007, I worked with a group of service users for the Mental Health Testimony Project. The project consisted of in-depth interviews from 50 long-term inmates of twentieth-century psychiatric institutions. My job was to manage the team to develop searchable keywords from the interviews for a database set up by Mental Health Media. These interviews are now archived in the British Library.

One of the volunteers working on the project said in response to the work:

> When you discover that someone has spent the better part of 40 years in an institution and left with no sense of the reason for their mental distress or recognition that this is something which could be discussed, it is difficult not to form the opinion that the system has potentially done more damage to their life than the circumstances which led them there initially.

My own response to analyzing the data was to write:

> I was surprised to read in such detail, and so many times over, the lives of people who experienced mental distress. It was obvious reading through so many case studies, that there was a pattern in people's experiences: of instability of family life, of employment, of relationships, of disharmony in external circumstances. How did we ever arrive at mental distress as being separate from our external lives? There are clear cases that we would now recognize whereby the triggers of distress were post-natal depression, or post traumatic shock disorder, that in those days were pathologized, the experients incarcerated, and institutionalized.

These personal testimonies clearly illustrated cases that an interviewee having a different point of view from their relative or a practitioner was in itself considered an indicator of mental illness. Do we do things differently today? In the new DSM-5, there is a category of 'oppositional defiant disorder' and of 'anosognosia' which means not recognizing you have an illness disorder.

Working on the Mental Health Testimony Project affected my understanding of the old style of psychiatric diagnosis and the treatment of mental health patients. I became biased against accepting without question the decisions of authority. The Testimony Project website with its clear, searchable triggers of social and economic stressors appeared to have gone offline in 2012. However, the original video recordings are still available at the British Library.

Why was the research data website no longer available? Was this due to financial pressures or was the data about personal difficulties and triggers of distress of those incarcerated too obvious? Did it not fit with the current consensus on the diseases of the brain model of mental health, even for a charity which supported those with mental health conditions? Has the consensus on the triggers of mental distress changed over the years or are they still well guarded?

The topic around mental health is so large that I have dedicated several chapters to it in Part Two. In them, I present data from my research with mental health practices in India and discuss contemporary western beliefs on spiritual interpretations of extreme experiences or breakdown.

SUMMARY

In this chapter, I have presented ways in which consensus and public opinion have changed in terms of issues that were assumed to be indicative of mental illness in the past. This included having a child outside of marriage, being a child born out of wedlock, being gay or lesbian or the acknowledgement of the various triggers of mental distress. It also included those who had been criminalized because of homosexual activity between consenting adults.

I also mentioned the topic of colonization, whereby settler populations decided that indigenous people were perhaps mentally challenged – this led to their offspring in Australia, Canada and the United States being removed from them for schooling, adoption and integration into white Christian culture. Then consensus changed, a cultural U-turn occurred, and compensation was considered.

These words form part of the apology by the Canadian Commission for Truth and Reconciliation (p.386):

Finally, we wish to apologize as well for our past dismissal of many of the riches of Native religious tradition. We broke some of your peace pipes and we considered some of your sacred practices as pagan and superstitious. This, too, had its origins in the colonial mentality, our European superiority complex which was grounded in a particular view of history. We apologize for this blindness and disrespect.

Communication strategies are considered later, as ways of determining and acknowledging a person's frameworks of knowledge. I have included people's beliefs about death and dying in the next chapters, as these specific beliefs seem to influence people's understandings of mental health.

PART TWO

8

CULTURAL KNOWLEDGE ON DEATH AND DYING

INTRODUCTION

This chapter describes a variety of beliefs about death and dying possessed by different ethnic and religious groups. Understanding societal beliefs about death is important because consensus about ritual practices is not constant or uniform throughout the world. With changing times, there are cultural U-turns happening as we understand more about other people's beliefs and practices.

It is important to consider the cultural variables in beliefs about death, as these often influence people's interpretations of their physical and mental wellbeing. This is key to grasping the interpretation of the symptoms of spiritual or extreme experiences, or mental health.

I will provide a brief overview of various ancient books of the dead which advise people on how to go about their lives during their final hours. Hindu and Muslim cultural and religious practices are also mentioned. Using the case study of Nelson Mandela, I will illustrate rituals carried out on his death in Africa.

This material was used when I taught seminars on death and dying in hospitals and medical schools. I explored the more recent professionalization and medicalization of death in the western world and noted that there was a taboo around death in the West. This meant that corpses were often hidden from view, although some societies always laid out their dead for viewing.

Case studies from India and Africa will be presented, illustrating conscious dying rituals, where people feel their time to die is present, their circle of life has come around and they withdraw quietly. Other societies pay attention to the soul and spirit after death, concepts that are mentioned in more detail in the following chapter.

Occasionally there are problems with defining death, and there are rare incidents of mistaken identification. This chapter also covers differences in bereavement that may occur in cases of sudden death or expected death. I offer some insight into the topic of sudden death and its effect on the living.

In Chapter 10, I will mention near-death and end-of-life experiences and bereavement apparitions. Here, however, I will explore different societies' beliefs about death and dying, followed in the next chapter with people's beliefs about survival beyond death.

When I facilitated seminars with frontline medical and healthcare staff on death and dying, I asked participants what they believed, and there appeared to be very little consensus about what happened after death. Staff may have had the same or similar clinical training but they were surprised to discover their beliefs about existential reality were often different.

Beliefs that an individual does not die with the human body were widespread. They included beliefs that ancestors continue to exert influence over their living relatives, or that there is a soul or spirit that moves on; or that *djinn* are discarnate entities which influence the health and wellbeing of living people. These beliefs in particular influence people's interpretations of their symptoms of mental distress or their extreme experiences. People's beliefs also influence their preferred treatment at the end of life, and whether or not they prepare living wills. Custom and practice in medical care at the end of life are being questioned and awareness is growing about doctors who choose different ways to die (O'Neil 2015).

In this chapter, I will touch on topics that some readers may be sensitive about – for example, if you have experienced a recent bereavement or a death that has been difficult to come to terms with. This might include the unexpected or disturbing death of a patient, colleague, close friend or relative, or any other death witnessed which is of significance. If you as a reader are recently bereaved, then do please read this section with caution.

It is important to study beliefs about survival beyond death because beliefs influence a patient's expectations of the medical and healthcare practices carried out during dying and after death; staff beliefs may influence the treatment they offer; migrant populations do not simply leave their beliefs at the point of entry to the UK (this is relevant even for subsequent generations); beliefs inform people's explanatory models for mental distress and may inhibit access to statutory services. Our beliefs may influence the ways we interact with patients and relatives. If a member of staff doesn't share the beliefs of patients and carers about death and dying, they may need to explore strategies to acknowledge them and eliminate conflicts that can arise.

My seminars with frontline staff who worked on a daily basis with dying patients indicated that not everyone had automatic access to counselling or supervision. In some areas of the UK, healthcare staff were well supported with appropriate supervision, but in other areas medical and healthcare practitioners seem to lack support. It seemed that a clear policy of care for staff working with dying patients was not always practised. One participant explained to the group that, after certain deaths, 'I just go into my car and cry'.

The London borough of Redbridge has developed a booklet entitled *To Comfort Always*. This is an intercultural spiritual care directory for use by frontline service providers. It sets out the preferences of different cultural groups who live in the borough. It has advice on where to contact chaplains, what to do if a post mortem is required, and concerns about organ donation. It would be useful if other hospitals and hospices followed this template and produced a document or website relevant to their local populations.

PROFESSIONALIZATION AND MEDICALIZATION OF DEATH

Funeral practices have changed over time. In the early twentieth century, in a Yorkshire or Irish village, local people washed and laid out the body in their homes. Relatives watched over it, while family and friends visited and paid their final respects. The family themselves were the pall-bearers. However, by the late twentieth century, in the same villages, professional undertakers had taken control: they laid out the body and arranged the viewing and burial.

In the past it was the midwife's job to lay out dead, as well as caring for births: people believed that without the ancestors returning after death, it would not be possible to create new babies. However, as a result of the UK Midwives Act of 1902, women were forced to choose and they chose to be legally registered midwives of births. In other societies like in Papua New Guinea, it was specifically the task of women to be midwife both to the newly deceased and the new-born.

In the west, many people die within a hospital environment away from public view. Death became seen as a medical event which needed to be certified. It was considered to have a physical cause, rather than being an act of God. Undertaking was originally a side line of carpentry, until undertaking became professionalized in the late seventeenth century. Today, funeral directors provide a commercial service and control over events sometimes seems to have been taken away from dying people and their families.

The Western medical ideal has become to 'vanquish' premature death: early death is regarded as preventable and therefore under individual control. Death or a fatal accident before old age is regarded as a loss of control over one's body. Such deaths are no longer regarded as simple misfortunes and therefore it is often felt that someone must be held to account.

As humans we often feel the need to 'control' death. Dying, death and corpses become hidden away from everyday life (in hospices, hospitals and cemeteries). Images of corpses are often censored from media reporting of actual events involving deaths. The result is that many people go through life without ever witnessing a death or seeing a dead body.

A colleague I taught with, Dr Elizabeth Archer, conducted a brief review of some medical literature. She found that in the *Oxford Textbook of Medicine* 'death' appeared in *every* section, but there was no section or chapter heading about the meaning of death. There was no index entry for death in any standard medical textbooks or in texts on physiology and biochemistry. There was plenty of information on palliative care for the dying, but no discussion of the nature of death itself. In spite of this, there were many variables in what people considered to be the principles of a good death in the UK (Smith 2000).

ANCIENT BELIEFS ABOUT DEATH AND BEYOND

In many societies, the dead were considered as 'beings'. They remained active and could confer blessings on the living, or they could affect the fertility of women and crops. They had to be correctly propitiated, as people believed hierarchies of power continue beyond death. People believed the dead could influence the mental wellbeing of the living.

Human beings appear to devote a great deal of attention to trying to understand death and dying. It is important to raise awareness of this, given the multicultural population in the UK. For example, in the London borough of Harrow, according to the 2011 census, 31.9% of residents stated they were White–British, with 69.1% of residents coming from minority ethnic groups.

In this section I will explore different ways of dying using case studies from ancient books of the dead (Tibetan, Egyptian, Mayan) and more modern cultural and religious beliefs – Christian, Hindu, Dinka and Daur. I will explore the concepts of the good and the bad death and beliefs about its influences on the living. The ancient texts used are the Egyptian Book of the Dead, the Tibetan Book of the Dead, the Maya Book of the Dead and, in Christian Europe, the *Ars Moriendi* (the Art of Dying).

The Egyptian Book of the Dead (*Pert em hru*) consists of a collection of rolls of ancient inscribed papyri: texts that include prayers, incantations, hymns and magical formulae for treating the deceased, written over 5,000 years ago. It was a guide for surviving the underworld and gaining access to the afterlife. First produced around the third millennium BCE, it was used for kings, then by the nobility and prominent figures. Only later was life after death considered a possibility for common citizens.

The Tibetan Book of the Dead (*Bardo Thodol*) was a series of Buddhist writings from the eighth century CE which were based on older texts as a guide for the dying and the dead. Guru Padma-Sambhava wrote them and they illustrate a preoccupation with life after death and rituals to conduct the soul to the beyond safely. The texts were buried in hills of central Tibet and rediscovered by an incarnation of the author's disciples. They are intended to guide humans through experiences of consciousness after death, to support us during the interval between death and the next rebirth.

The Mayan Book of the Dead was gleaned from the Ceramic Codex, from funeral vases and pictures dating to around the eighth century CE. There were stories about the underworld and its inhabitants. When the Spanish arrived, they destroyed much of Mayan written material, produced on richly illustrated bark folded screens. Mayan beliefs about death were interpreted from ceramic vessels, painted in the same style as in the literature.

In medieval Christian Europe, the book of the dead was the *Ars Moriendi*, produced from the early fifteenth century CE onwards. These manuals informed the dying about what to expect and prescribed prayers, actions and attitudes that would lead to a 'good death' and salvation. The *Ars Moriendi* sets out Christian beliefs and practices concerning death, dying and the afterlife. It expanded on rites for priests visiting the sick into a manual for both clergy and laypeople. It was written to address the fundamental problem of human existence in the face of an impermanent life.

Dr Madeleine Gray, professor of Ecclesiastic History at the University of South Wales, has explained that in medieval times people were worried about 'judgement' and the need for 'mercy'. The medieval assumption was that a person needed the prayers of others to release them from purgatory. At that time they didn't appear to have a narrative of the soul or spirit beyond the body, or of reincarnation. It seemed death was feared, but prayers to saints like Saint Christopher would supposedly ensure a person would not die a bad or unpredictable death.

MODERN BELIEFS ABOUT DEATH: SOCIAL LIFE AND BEYOND
Beliefs from India

Cultural requirements around dying differ. For example, in Kolkata in India one psychiatrist, Dr Soumitra Basu, felt obliged to challenge the rules when it came to his own father's death.

> We have our own limitations and we can't only make decisions based on what we have studied. For example, I have been told to withhold hydration to a comatose patient to facilitate passive euthanasia, but what should I do? For me, giving water to my dying father was a very important thing in my life, one of my most cherished memories. The day my father was departing, I was able to give him a spoonful of water on his tongue. How can I take a decision that denies the same experience to others? (Tobert 2001, p.15)

I have undertaken many fieldwork trips to India where I learnt that active dying rituals were practised: these were known as a state of *samadhi*, which, through meditation, was the complete concentration and absorption of the consciousness of an individual at the time of death. A religious person would realize when it was their time to die so they would refuse all food and water and meditate until they passed away. This happened with H.H. Sri Chandrasekharendra Saraswati, the 68th Shankaracharya of Kanchipuram in Tamil Nadu, South India. He attained *samadhi* in 1994, aged 99 years old.

In contrast to this kind of conscious death, in Hindu India there were early practices whereby the wife of a royal or warrior caste man would immolate herself on the pyre of her husband. She did this because she believed that she would go through social death and exclusion if she remained alive. Although the custom of *sati* was banned in 1829, in practice it still occurs (though rarely) in twenty-first-century rural India.

There were also active dying rituals among Muslims which I learnt about when I visited the mosque at Nagore in India. There the saint Hazarath Sayed Mohamed Yousef (born in 1501 AD: 909h) was said to perform miracles, even as a foetus in the womb. At the site of Nagore mosque, when he left his body for the last time, his son recited prayers above his grave and the saint was heard to reply from the tomb. In 1570 a thatched roof was put over the grave, and as the flow of offerings and gifts began, walls were erected and then a domed roof was built above. Today there is a huge mosque on the site of the grave which people of all faiths attend for healing.

Death rituals for a Muslim have other requirements which are carried out in any part of the world: 'To Allah we belong, and to Him is our return' (Quran 2:156). 'Death is an important time in a Muslim's life because it is then they continue their spiritual advancement. Death is the pinnacle of a person's religious journey.' Upon death 'the person's eyes are closed and their jaw is secured shut. It is a religious requirement that the body be ritually washed and draped before burial, which should be as soon as possible after death' (Saleha).

Beliefs from Africa

Among the Dinka of Sudan in Africa, the anthropologist Lienhardt (1990) has reported similar activities for holy men or diviners. When an honoured elder holy man chose an active death, his relatives dug a burial pit within the cattle byre. He was aware his faculties were passing. His eyes were dim and his teeth were falling out so he told the people of his lineage that he wished to be buried alive. He was laid out on a wooden bed, lowered into the grave and then hymns were sung by those attending. Women and children were sent away but the men stayed to hear the buried man's prophesies. Once the master no longer responded to those present, they covered the grave and constructed a shrine over it. They did not say 'Alas, he is dead!' They said 'it is very good' (1990, p.302) or 'the master has gone to the earth' (1990, p.314).

Among the Nuer peoples, if a man dies without offspring, there will be a ghost marriage (Evans-Pritchard 1940). His kinsman will marry and have children in his name. If the brother wants children of his own, he must be able to afford a second wife.

When I was working in Darfur in Sudan, a photo of a dead Fur person was believed to capture their soul. When I showed villagers photos including a person who had died the previous year, the face of the deceased was blocked out and removed from that photo so their soul could move about freely.

DEATH OF NELSON MANDELA

Death rituals were publically seen to support the spirit and soul when Nelson Mandela died on 5 December 2013. He was South Africa's first African president and was inaugurated in 1994. There were ten days of mourning after his death. During the funeral service his coffin lay on a carpet of cow skins. This Xhosa chief from the Thembu clan called Madiba was buried in his home village of Qunu, his coffin covered with a leopard skin.

To achieve spiritual harmony, people believed his soul needed to be reunited at burial with his mortal remains. If this had not occurred, the spirit might wander restlessly and cause misfortune to his family. People believed that the ritual return pleased the ancestors, appeased the creator and protected the family.

As Nelson Mandela's body was transported home by plane, his grandson performed the rituals required to invoke his spirit's return. This involved speaking to the body during its journey back to the place of its birth, guiding its living spirit by talking about the names of rivers and lands during the flight and informing it when the body it inhabited was to be buried. Songs of praise of the family and the lineage group were invoked, as were deceased ancestors, with whom Mandela would be reunited.

An ox was slaughtered, and if it bellowed during slaughter, this would be taken as a sign the ancestors were pleased and welcomed the newly deceased. Those present would share and eat the meat. A traditional poet introduced Mandela to the ancestors. Rain during funeral ceremonies was also taken to mean that the spirit and ancestral world welcomed the deceased.

The house of the family was cleansed with herbs to release any attachment the deceased might have there. After a period of mourning (one year), another ox was slaughtered and the mourning clothes themselves were burnt. Even after the funeral, ceremonies would be held to invoke Mandela's spirit, inviting him to mediate between the living and the creator.

Beliefs from Asia: China, Manchuria, Thailand

In China, the dead are traditionally buried and not cremated. People believe that incorrect funeral procedures may negatively influence the family of the deceased. Those who attend do not wear the colour red and all mirrors are covered (as they were in Victorian houses of mourning). Within Mahayana Buddhism, the intermediate time between death and rebirth is called *bardo*, an important time which can influence the next rebirth. It is for this reason that relatives must undertake appropriate prayers and remembrance ceremonies. In this way, the deceased can expect a more positive rebirth.

In Northern Manchuria, the Daur Mongols (Humphrey 1996) were farmers who grew grains, fished, herded animals and hunted. Upon death they believed a person changed into an ancestral spirit. Death transformed the souls of certain people into spirits which became free from physical human bodies and were able to reside in other objects in nature (rocks or trees).

Shamans may be buried in hollowed-out tree trunks: bark was replaced so the tree could continue to grow. In death, shamans were linked to specific places in the landscape: a deceased shaman's body was placed on a hill-top scaffold, the bones later collected for burial. The landscape became the location for spirits of ancestral shamans as these places were designated the focus of future rituals. Topics on ancestral spirits are considered in the following chapter.

My colleague, the German doctor Andreas Winkelmann, conducted medical anthropology research in an anatomy laboratory in Thailand. He discovered that the cadavers of dead people were social beings, known respectfully by medical students as the 'Great Teacher'. He reported on laboratory social rituals in Thailand where there was a dedication ceremony and prayers before medical processes began to introduce students to cadavers. Medical students called bodies in the anatomy lab by their actual social names in life and referred to them as the Great Teacher which was an indication of the high social position of cadavers (Winkelmann and Güldner 2004).

Contemporary medical doctors in the UK remember saying prayers of thanks as students before beginning dissection and at the end of the year they attended a service of thanks at a local church or cathedral. One doctor, Lauren Gavaghan, said: 'at Newcastle, there was a lovely service of thanks with the families of those who had donated their bodies also present. It was very emotional actually, though the families seemed to take something from it, knowing that they were respecting their loved ones' wishes to be used after death in this way, to further medical students understanding and learning' (personal comment).

DEFINITION OF BIOLOGICAL DEATH...?

In the West, there used to be a discussion about the definition of 'death' (Zamperetti et al. 2003). Signs within the body used to be 'loss of heartbeat' or 'loss of breath', a lack of sensitivity to electrical stimuli or coldness or rigor mortis. 'Brainstem death' meant an individual's body could not recover independent function. However, did 'brain dead' mean the body was dead? Could a body still breathe or be in a persistent vegetative state (PVS) and be brain dead?

For a while, it seemed that the definition of 'dead' depended on the intention for the corpse (Evans 1996, p.135). A cadaver might be kept 'alive' using machinery, so its organs could be harvested directly and transplanted into a recipient patient. Signs of death such as loss of heartbeat or breathing were masked or hidden by the effects of the life-support technology and the individual continued to 'look alive'. Transplant surgeons who wanted to use organs from cadavers turned off machines and waited to ensure the donor didn't breathe on their own.

In the UK the Liverpool Care Pathway (LCP) was set up for dying patients and covered palliative care options for patients in their final days or hours of life.[1] Guidelines were developed to help members of a multidisciplinary team of hospital doctors and nurses give the same kind of high-quality end-of-life care that terminally ill patients received in a hospice. The system, which may involve the withdrawal

---

1   www.endoflifecare.nhs.uk/care-pathway/step-5-care-in-the-last-days-of-life/liverpool-care-pathway.aspx

of medication, food and fluids and increased comfort, was developed in the 1990s during collaboration between the Royal Liverpool University Hospital and the Marie Curie hospice to provide a model of best practice.

However, critics labelled it the 'road to death' and those who feared abuse accused the NHS of killing off elderly patients. In contrast, supporters said relatives on the programme had a peaceful and dignified death. The Royal College of Physicians found nearly half the families involved were not informed of clinical decisions to put their relative on the pathway. The LCP was phased out in 2013/14. The NHS National End-of-Life programme came to a close, but the NHS produced a guide for carers and those nearing the end of life entitled *Actions for End-of-Life Care* to support people living with long-term conditions.

We need to explore the complexity of defining death. In the UK, there appeared to be a dilemma over the definition of death. There did not appear to be a single, clear, universally understood and accepted term for death. There seemed to be degrees of death, with different tissues in the same body 'dying' at different rates.

SUDDEN DEATH AND BEREAVEMENT

Expected death and sudden death produce very different social responses and bereavement experiences for those who have lost a loved one. In the UK and Ireland in 2015, 6,000 people a year committed suicide, around 1,500 women and 4,500 men, according to the Samaritans.[2] The number of young men committing suicide has increased over the past few decades. There are complex factors which lead a person to take their own life.

Rarely is there one single trigger – there may be an important 'last straw'. Other factors include physical illness (acute and chronic), alcohol and drug abuse, social isolation, housing, money and job problems. The final straw may be the end of an important relationship, debt or a court case, losing one's home or job or a deeply emotional event.

At least 140,000 people in England and Wales attempt suicide every year: this number is rising among young people. Single men and

---

2   www.samaritans.org/news/samaritans-urges-men-talk-about-their-problems

women, never married, divorced or widowed, are much more likely to commit suicide. The act itself is not acceptable to many faiths and faith itself appeared to reduce the risk of suicide. People with strong religious beliefs tended to have more supportive social networks. A failed suicide may be a 'cry for help', common among teenage girls, but it occurs in both sexes. It's a mistake not to take it seriously.

Losing someone suddenly is intensely painful, but with intentional death there are difficult issues to work through for loved ones, friends and colleagues. During the grieving process, the bereaved often ask agonizing questions and search for explanations. Common feelings (as well as sadness and bereavement) may include guilt for not recognizing the problem and anger at the person who killed themselves.

Faith, pressure and suicide

There may be additional fears if parents of a certain faith have a gay son. For example, with Muslim parents, if family and friends are aware they have a gay son, they may fear losing everything. They may become social outcasts, not only from the community but from their own extended family in the UK and in their country of ancestral origin.

Other children in the family may be shunned, unable to get jobs in their community or unable to marry as their blood may be considered to be tainted. It may lead to gay Muslims being forced into a loveless marriage, experiencing depression, homelessness, drug abuse or suicide. Being Asian, male and gay can be a cause of pressure: suicide is forbidden, as is homosexuality. It is a taboo subject: most men never publicly admit to being gay and they have fear being ostracized or forced into marriage to protect their family reputation.

The Home Office Forced Marriage Unit gives advice and support related to forced marriage, and 14% of those who approach the unit are men. The unit receives over 80 reports about male victims, with many cases linked to sexuality. In the majority of cases, families are from South Asia, Pakistan, India and Bangladesh. However, the numbers may be under-reported: figures may be below the actual number of forced marriages. Victims, usually aged between 15 and 24, may be locked up, subjected to physical violence or forcibly removed to other countries if they refuse to comply with family wishes.

SUMMARY

This chapter has covered a variety of beliefs about death and dying of different ethnic and religious groups. I have noted the importance of understanding cultural variables, as beliefs about death often influence people's beliefs about their physical and mental wellbeing. I have given an overview of the more recent medicalization of death in the western world and the professionalization of those who deal with funerals.

I also briefly presented various ancient books of the dead which advised people how to go about their lives and live during their last hours. I offered insight into the topic of sudden death and its effect on bereavement in the living. Examples were given from India and Africa of conscious dying rituals where people felt their time had come and they withdrew to die. I noted that death and corpses were often hidden from view in the west. Using the case of Nelson Mandela, I illustrated the rituals carried out on death.

Some areas in the UK had good documentary and interpersonal support for medical and healthcare practitioners, but other frontline staff seemed to lack support. What steps could be taken to ensure hospital staff of all grades are aware of different religious rituals performed on death and are themselves supported? Some hospitals situated within a multicultural population have developed protocols for those coping with death and the required rituals.

Are cultural and religious death rituals always considered important? In some medical schools, prayers are held at the end of term for those who gave their bodies to the anatomy lab. In the following chapter I consider people's beliefs about survival beyond death.

9

CULTURAL BELIEFS ABOUT SURVIVAL BEYOND DEATH

There is something infinitely healing in the repeated refrains of nature,
the assurance that dawn comes after night, and spring after winter

Rachel Carson

INTRODUCTION: CULTURAL KNOWLEDGE

When I facilitated seminars at healthcare centres as part of cultural equalities training, I used to ask colleagues about their beliefs regarding what happened after death. I invited them to explore what kinds of beliefs co-existed in the room. I found that although people had the same or similar clinical training, they often had quite different views about reality, depending on their religion or their personal spiritual beliefs. For some reason, this wide range of beliefs seemed to surprise participants.

For years, a linear model was most useful for describing the general assumption that life began at conception or birth and continued until death, which was the end of the process. This section explores cultural beliefs about what happens after death and the implications for those who remain: it offers a forum for discussion about cultural understandings.

The model involving 'ashes to ashes and dust to dust' is not ubiquitous in human existence. In the west, one part of the population believed there was no survival beyond death, only mundane physicality, while those who claimed to be psychics, mediums or clairvoyants asserted consciousness survived beyond bodily death. The psychologist

Charles Tart (1997) has said that we long assumed our thoughts, feelings and emotions were simply brain reactions that dissolved with the brain upon death. Now there is a different awareness.

Some people believe that we only live once and that death is a full stop. Others believe that we live once, die and then go to heaven or hell. Yet others believe humans are born, live a bit, die and reincarnate repeatedly. There appears to be no consensus on this matter.

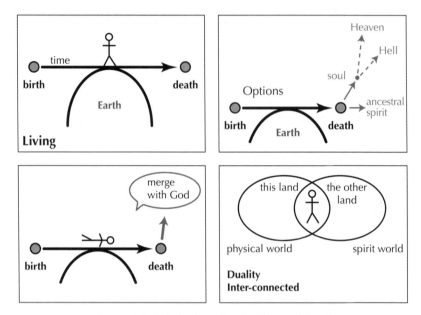

Figure 9.1. Beliefs about Survival beyond Death

This chapter covers cultural beliefs from different societies and looks at reincarnation beliefs. I present the thoughts of the Swiss psychiatrist Elizabeth Kübler-Ross about dying and those of the Indian seer and philosopher Sri Aurobindo. I set out death rituals from India – these rituals are supposed to ensure the safe passage of the ancestors.

I also present evidence from psychiatrists like Ian Stevenson, which is suggestive of reincarnation, and also from a GP, who suggests it is normal for bereaved people to experience a presence or vision of their deceased partners. This material seems to cause one to ask: what data is veridical and according to whom?

Cultural beliefs that an individual did not die with the human body when it died have been widespread. They include beliefs that ancestors continue to exert influence over their living relatives and must be correctly prayed for, or that *djinn* were discarnate beings which influenced living people's mental health.

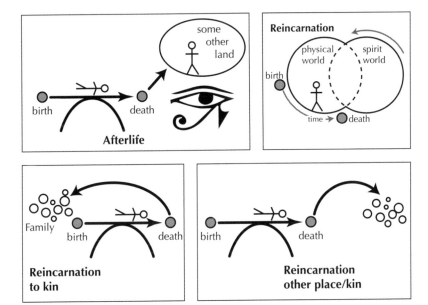

Figure 9.2. Beliefs about the Afterlife

I explore cultural knowledge and beliefs about what happens during and after physical death and beliefs about the survival and continuity of consciousness beyond death. There are beliefs from different world societies on rebirth and reincarnation and there are anomalous experiences people have when they care for the soul and spirit of the deceased. I explore various cultures' belief systems concerning consciousness after death, extra-corporeal perception and ancestral spirits. Beliefs about this may influence clinical responses to patients.

I will also consider material from Stevenson on his research on memories of reincarnation, the work of Dewi Rees on spouse returnees and material from Jean-Guy Goulet on Canadian native peoples. This material is important because a medical or healthcare professional's personal beliefs about death might influence their conduct and communication with patients regarding end-of-life decisions, advance directives, religious rituals and potential treatment or the withdrawal of such.

I ask whether our understanding of the nature of physical reality and consciousness after death influences our judgement, notably with regard to certain medical matters. Do our beliefs about consciousness beyond death influence our frameworks for understanding issues relating to mental health?

There used to be the assumption that when the body died, the soul departed. To explore this, an experiment was set up by Dr MacDougal of Massachusetts General Hospital in 1906; he had the hypothesis that the human soul had mass. He set up an experiment to weigh the bodies of dying patients to see if any weight loss occurred in death by the soul departing. His results were inconclusive.

In 2014, the skeleton of a Siberian woman was found whom the elders considered was linked to the wellbeing of the living – in their wisdom, they decided to rebury this ancient female mummified corpse. As an ancestor, she was considered to be present and active, influencing the lives of the living. There are many narratives about death and survival but we do not know which ones are truths and which are beliefs. It probably depends on the beliefs of the reader or observer.

BELIEFS ABOUT SURVIVAL BEYOND DEATH AND MENTAL HEALTH

People's beliefs about survival beyond death do influence their interpretation of mental health symptoms. I have worked in the borough of Harrow, which was the ninth most ethnically diverse local authority in England and Wales, with over 40 different ethnicities. One third of Harrow's residents were born abroad. Local medical and healthcare workers were aware of different models of human existence.

During a needs assessment project (Tobert 2008) with BAME communities in North West London, community members explained that religion, faith and stories about migration were important to mental wellbeing and should be considered part of mental health promotion. The report on this mental health promotion project is available (Tobert 2010a).

Community leaders in Harrow helped healthcare staff understand that beliefs about death were important for understanding the ways people interpreted symptoms of distress and mental ill health. Many different ethnic groups believed that an individual did not die with the human body. There were widespread beliefs that ancestors continued to exert influence over their living relatives, and that *djinn* were discarnate beings which influenced living people's mental health. In some societies, a human being was believed to consist of both physical and non-physical components, some of which preceded and survived death.

In many non-western countries, much human misfortune and mental ill health have been attributed to the ghosts of those who died an untimely death. For example, belief in ghosts was ubiquitous in Asia and rural Africa and with first generation Asian migrants. A ghost required prayers in order to become an ancestor and be recycled and reborn as a baby. Conception occurred through the regeneration of an ancestral soul and this resulted in cultural concerns about having a 'good' death so ancestors reincarnated and did not remain in limbo like ghosts to trouble the mental health of the living.

The book *Talking with the Spirits* by Jack Hunter and David Luke (2014) presented various examples from the UK, the Amazon, Singapore and Taiwan where mediums communicated with beings in spirit. People's beliefs about survival beyond death were important: they influenced a patient's expectations of medical and healthcare practices. This was relevant even for subsequent generations. People's beliefs informed the way they explained mental distress and in some cases inhibited their access to statutory services. Cultural beliefs about what happened after death had implications for the mental health of those who remained.

DEATH RITUALS AND REINCARNATION
South Indian Rituals

On one of my visits to Rameshwaram in South India, I saw that rituals for the dead were carried out in public and in sacred places. The seashore was a healing place for prayers for the dead, for rituals conducted for mental peace and closure after bereavement. This town was said to be located at one of four energy points in India which held that sub-continent's soul. Thousands of pilgrims bathed in the sea each day at sunrise.

On the shore one day, a freelance pundit sat cross-legged under an umbrella, attended by three brothers with shaved heads, one holding a dark brown ceramic pot with a lid containing ashes. Prayer rituals for their dead relative were conducted on the seashore: the eldest son took a pot of ashes upon his head and was followed by his brothers. He walked into sea, as far as he could go, and then gifted the ceramic pot and its contents into the waters, followed by garlands of fresh flowers. As the flowers drifted into the ocean, the brothers stood still in prayer. Then they loosened their white dhoti, allowing the sea to take them and then submerged themselves completely under the water.

Pilgrims in India have explained that the physical body enveloped an ethereal body. After death, cremation destroyed the first body, liberating the second ethereal body into the ether. Offerings of rice balls were made to protect the ethereal body with an outer case during its journey to the abode of the ancestors. Once at the abode of the ancestors, the protective case was sloughed off and the ethereal body would experience the consequences of past actions.

In India, people said a person consisted of a body, breath and a soul, and identity was not fixed at the skin. A living person's body appeared to be permeable to the spirits of the dead. People claimed there was good and bad death and good and bad spirits of the dead. People who died a 'good' death were cremated, resulting in rebirth and renewal. Those who died a 'bad' death were blocked from being reborn. Much human misfortune was attributed to the ghosts of those who had died an untimely death.

People were concerned about having a 'good death'. The anthropologist Jonathan Parry (1994) did fieldwork in Banaras city, famous for dealing with death. Pilgrims went to the banks of the River Ganges to cremate their loved ones, where they were led through the ceremonies by priests and pundits. The aim of post-cremation rites was to convert the ghost of a deceased relative into an ancestor to help them achieve the journey to their final resting place and to ensure the deceased achieved 'a good state' (sadgati) after death. This was as important for Hindus in Manchester as it was in Manhattan or Mumbai.

Among Indian populations, there were other concepts – like karma – which influenced rebirth and reincarnation. Jain devotees from India claimed all actions, good or bad, attached karmic matter to our soul. Evil actions were heavier and harder to get rid of. Liberation came either by preventing karma by abandoning action or by living a life of austerity to release any attached karma. Hindu followers believed karma was a moral law of cause and effect whereby the actions of one life were carried over into the next and determined not only a person's fate, but also those of their kin. A person's actions had consequences meriting reward or punishment, as did those of their kin. Buddhist people believed good or evil deeds in one life were rewarded or punished in the next. By adhering to the correct path, humans could break the chains of karma and achieve enlightenment.

BELIEFS OF AN INDIAN SAGE

While in India, I visited the ashram of Sri Aurobindo where he wrote a great deal about the soul's journey after death. He was a philosopher who had spent the greater part of his life in Pondicherry, South India, although he had studied as a child in the UK. He devoted his life to the study of consciousness. His writings were influential both in India and among western populations. He propounded the following:

> at the time of death the being goes out of the body through the head; it goes out in the subtle body and goes to different planes of existence for a short time until it has gone through certain experiences which are the result of its earthly existence. Afterwards it reaches the psychic world where it rests in a kind of sleep, until it is time for it to start a new life on earth. (Sri Aurobindo, p.431)

He wrote:

> The soul takes birth each time, and each time a mind, life and body are formed out of the materials of universal nature according to the soul's past evolution and its need for the future.... The soul gathers the essential elements of its experiences in life and makes that its basis of growth in the evolution; when it returns to birth it takes up with its mental, vital, physical sheaths so much of its Karma as is useful to it in the new life for further experience. (p.134)

BELIEFS OF AN AMERICAN PSYCHIATRIST

The Swiss American psychiatrist, Elizabeth Kübler-Ross (1969), had a very spiritual outlook on life and death. She pioneered insights into death and dying and had visited a concentration camp on the outskirts of Poland. When she taught medical students, she used case studies of terminally ill patients so the students could face and respond to live patients.

Later in her life, she became interested in out-of-body experiences and mediumship. She is quoted as saying:

after your death, when most of you for the first time realize what life here is all about, you will begin to see that your life here is almost nothing, but the sum total of every choice you have made during every moment of your life. Your thoughts, which you are responsible for, are as real as your deeds. You will begin to realize that every word and every deed affects your life and has also touched thousands of lives (Kübler-Ross 1969).

Her last book (1998) was her autobiography The Wheel of Life where she wrote:

For those who seek to understand it, death is a highly creative force. The highest spiritual values of life can originate from the thought and study of death. Watching a peaceful death of a human being reminds us of a falling star; one of a million lights in a vast sky that flares up for a brief moment only to disappear into the endless night forever.

CROSS-CULTURAL REINCARNATION BELIEFS

For many years there was an assumption that the only people to hold beliefs about reincarnation were the Hindu peoples from South Asia. Many scholars took it for granted that India was the home of rebirth beliefs, with accompanying concepts of karma and the cycle of reward, punishment and salvation. However, India was only one place of many to hold this belief. Obeyesekere (1981), a professor of anthropology at Princeton University, has argued that beliefs in reincarnation were also central to Native Americans, Africans and Oceanic peoples.

The anthropologists Mills and Slobodin (1994) have suggested that the concept of reincarnation could not be 'brought into line' with western scholars' understandings and so they neglected the study of it. Their colleague, Goulet (1994), was a professor of anthropology in Ottawa, Canada and he conducted research amongst the NaDene Tha of Northern Alberta, who considered themselves Roman Catholic.

They claimed the souls of individuals who had died sought to be reborn. The relatives would ask that the soul of the deceased be guided back into a womb. Of the 41 cases noted by the author, 18 had changed gender. Identification was a gradual process involving other people's recollections of a child's past life, and this information became part of a child's own sense of identity.

The NaDene Tha consider sexual intercourse as necessary but not sufficient for human reproduction. The indication that a reincarnation is imminent has certain signs: someone may have a dream announcing the birth; there may be visions of the dead person roaming around; a young child may have recollections of the individual he or she was in previous life; others may notice similarities of personality and habits; or, there may be birthmarks which relate to the previous incarnation.

Young and Goulet (1994) have claimed that in recent years anthropologists have expressed sympathy with 'non-rational' ways of thinking and with people's anomalous experiences. However, they also suggested scholars rarely acknowledged different beliefs as veridical. Their book challenges a western rationalist bias and takes other cultures' beliefs more seriously than in the past. Goulet and Young (1994) also explored what happened to anthropologists when confronted by irreconcilable differences and extraordinary events experienced during fieldwork which did not fit with their western rationalist approach.

EVIDENCE SUGGESTIVE OF SURVIVAL BEYOND DEATH

What evidence is there of survival beyond death? Does it come from end-of-life experiences that some patients report just before death or the bereavement visions of those who have experienced the loss of a loved one? Could evidence come from the reincarnation memories that some claim to have or from the memories of those who have had organ transplants? Are those who claim skills of mediumship providers of evidence?

End-of-life experiences

I wonder whether the end-of-life experiences mentioned in Chapter 11 are suggestive of survival beyond death. Peter Fenwick was a neuro-psychiatrist who recorded death-bed phenomena (Fenwick and Fenwick 2008). He conducted research into end-of-life experiences. Sometimes he said people dying needed to talk about and acknowledge the process: they may experience a life review or visions of pre-deceased relatives or pets. The dying may or may not report these experiences which many find calming. There are more details about his work and that of his colleagues in Chapter 11.

Bereavement experiences: sense of presence

Are bereavement experiences suggestive of survival beyond death? In a study by Dewi Rees, a GP and medical director of a hospice in Birmingham, some people felt a sense of presence after bereavement. In the 1970s he studied widows and widowers who experienced a sense of presence of their deceased spouse. Many people found the experience helpful; it was as though 'a continuing relationship exists between the living and the dead' (1971, p.37).

In the past, doctors were not told about such revelations since one ran the risk of being certified insane. Freud dismissed bereavement presences as psychotic hallucinations and some clergy considered them contrary to doctrinal belief. But what do we believe today? Is the mounting evidence of visionary experiences suggestive that they are veridical? Is a felt presence an apparition or a delusion? The Hearing Voices Network has suggested that the phenomena were normal after bereavement (Intervoice).

Dewi Rees published a paper in the *British Medical Journal* on his bereaved patients' visionary experiences (1970). He wrote: '50 per cent of widowed people have experiences of this type, and that these experiences are normal and helpful.' Around 50% of the 295 respondents had it and many considered it a 'religious experience'. About 39% of widowed people had 'a sense of the presence of the deceased': 14% saw them, 12% heard and spoke to them and 3% felt physically touched. The experiences were not sought but occurred spontaneously.

With regard to the presences of the deceased, Dewi suggested in a letter to the *Church Times* that 'This type of experience is common and has important theological implications, yet is almost completely disregarded by the Church' (1970, p.37). He asked why the Church accepted that Christ had lived but assumed perceptions of the bereaved had no basis in reality. He wondered why one was accepted and the other denied. He claimed his results have been replicated at least twice in the USA 'with almost identical findings'. In other surveys on the subject of presences, the percentage was 47% to 63%.

Apparitions or delusions?

The Society for Psychical Research was founded in the UK in 1882[1] to systematically study apparitions and publish scholarly reports on the research. The first study of 17,000 respondents was called a 'census of hallucinations' and was published in 1886. People reported sounds, touch, smell and temperature changes, although at other times there might just be an overwhelming 'sense of presence'. The perception could be of a short duration and it was usually perceived while the person was awake.

Various explanations have been given over time: apparitions were said to be different from projections, by a person's mind, of a deceased person. They might be said to be hallucinations if only one person perceived them. However, if more than one person perceived them, they might be considered to be mass delusions or real apparitions (depending on the beliefs and interpretation of the observer).

Our belief system about the end of life and our fear of death appears to define and influence our judgement of those who experience extreme experiences. Psychiatrists became interested in the topic but did this have anything to do with reincarnation?

Reincarnation, memory and birthmarks

Ian Stevenson was a professor of psychiatry at the University of Virginia, Charlottesville. Born in 1918, he trained in medicine then specialized in psychiatry and became particularly interested in researching evidence suggestive of reincarnation. He claimed that the birthmarks he studied were suggestive of survival beyond death. His books have been said to be the most scientific to date on the subject (1997).

Stevenson noticed a pattern in the case studies: usually a child was young, between the ages of two and four. They told their parents of a past life and had unusual behaviour patterns: the child often asked to be taken to places of a previous existence. However, he found that after the age of five, behaviour patterns and memories faded. He obtained witnesses, cross-checked statements of informants and claimed his cases could be explained as being 'suggestive of reincarnation'.

---

1   www.spr.ac.uk/page/history-society-psychical-research-parapsychology

He presented an analysis of the results: 225 case studies where people were born with birthmarks or defects and they claimed these related to past lives or the manner of past deaths. Informants claimed their birthmarks related to their past death experience. He selected birthmarks rather than any other kind of memory since he considered they provided an objective kind of evidence. He recorded behavioural memories and phobias which may have been related to a mode of death in a previous life; people remembered violent deaths in 51% of cases.

Stevenson recorded one case of a boy in Turkey, where birthmarks resembled an original remembered wound. He traced the medical certificate of the recalled past-life person. He recorded one child who remembered being killed by a blow to back of head, who was born with a depressed occipital part of his skull on which there was a birthmark. In recalled cases of shooting in a previous life, Stevenson recorded birthmarks which corresponded to a bullet wound in the head. Wounds were verified against the size and location of the birthmark. Some children who remembered mutilations were born with the corresponding limb missing.

Stevenson suggested there was some kind of memory transmitted between lives, some kind of karmic replay. He proposed reincarnation as the most suitable explanation. I wonder how we might respond to Stevenson's physical birthmark examples and how this material fits with our own beliefs about reality and extreme experiences. Antonia Mills was a colleague of Stevenson and she wrote an interesting article on alternative suggestions for children's nightmares (1994) – that they were recalling things from past lives.

Organ transplant and memory

In the west there was sometimes a dilemma over the definition of death. A cadaver may be kept 'alive' using machinery so organs can be harvested directly from its body and transplanted into the recipient patient. Many cultures have been slow to accept the use of organ transplants. There may, however, be other issues concerning beliefs about organ memory.

An interesting article was published on memories from donor body organs which influenced the wellbeing and behaviour of recipients (NAMAH 2016). There were some anecdotes collected that may challenge our beliefs.

There was also the narrative about body cells possibly retaining some kind of memory or consciousness. Paul Pearsall (1998) was an American psycho-neuro immunologist who collected the testimonies of heart transplant patients who believed their organs retained memories of the donor. One of his more unusual stories was about an eight-year-old girl who received the heart of a murdered ten-year-old and then had such disturbing nightmares that her mother took her to a psychiatrist. Based on the girl's descriptions, her mother and the psychiatrist eventually went to the police who found and convicted the donor's murderer.

But was it the cells of the heart which retained memory or did the recipient receive information by telepathy (from the deceased)? Or did the donor's spirit overshadow (or take possession of) the recipient? How could organ memory occur? Was the story fabricated? Pearsall provides other narratives in his book. Could these be evidence of the survival of consciousness beyond death?

As medical and healthcare providers, how would we respond if a patient reported narratives about donor memory? The explanatory model we choose would depend on our belief system about the nature of human existence, influenced by the common consensus view of our cultural background. Our belief systems influence how we interpret symptoms of mental distress and the ways we treat extreme experiences.

PRE-NATAL ANCESTRAL MEMORIES

In order to broaden the multiple ways of understanding distress, in this section I will consider studies that explore intergenerational triggers for trauma, which occur to one generation, but influence another. I will look at those who have claimed to have had ancestral memories which disturbed them. Authors like Bruce Lipton and Gabor Mate have spoken about the influences of a traumatic childhood on the mental health of an adult; likewise, a recent paper has shown an association between psychosis of poverty and being fostered/adopted (Longden et al. 2015). Another paper has explored links between auditory hallucinations and the stressors of being a migrant with a broken sense of self and the pain of losing everything (Rhodes et al. 2015). However, I will explore those who claim to have experienced trauma beyond the person.

Intergenerational transmission of trauma

Epigenetics is the study of body cells influenced by external or environmental factors (beyond the genes). Bruce Lipton is an American biologist who has said that 'We now know that we influence the activity of our genes by our actions, perceptions, beliefs and attitudes' (2014a). A mother's perception of the world influences the genetic makeup of her child, as stress hormones pass into the placenta. He believes that 'genes and DNA can be manipulated by our beliefs', He is not the only brilliant mind to propose such a mind-bending idea. In fact, he says that our DNA and cells do not control our health; rather our emotions do: our state of consciousness could influence our body and this could be passed on to children (Lipton 2014b).

However, the physician Gabor Mate questions genetics as a cause of mental illness. He suggests mental illness, addiction and most chronic illnesses are linked to childhood loss and trauma (Cassani 2013). His perspective is interesting, although psychiatrists I interviewed for the book *Spiritual Psychiatries* also suggested that there may also be other profound spiritual influences on mental wellbeing which go beyond birth and childhood and included past lives and karma (Tobert 2014).

In New York, a study has found that Nazi Holocaust trauma in one generation was passed on to the next generation through the genes. This was the theory of epigenetic inheritance: environmental factors which could affect the genes of a person's children. 'Genetic changes stemming from the trauma suffered by Holocaust survivors are capable of being passed on to their children, the clearest sign yet that one person's life experience can affect subsequent generations' (Thomson 2015). Studies illustrated that post-traumatic stress disorder and trauma could occur across generations, from people who had direct experiences of them to their offspring.

The America journalist, Judith Shulevitz, has written about research involving case studies with Nazi Holocaust survivors, indigenous Americans and people who experienced the Cambodian civil war (2014). She reported on Rachel Yehuda's research on the intergenerational transmission of trauma through memory, biology and culture.

Yehuda studied the children of Holocaust survivors and those of pregnant women who survived the attack on the World Trade Centre in 2001. The descendants of those who experienced the Nazi Holocaust had altered stress hormones which may predispose them to anxiety (Yehuda *et al.* 2005, 2015).

In Israel at the University of Haifa, a psychology course was offered on the memory of the Holocaust where participants studied how traumatic experiences could be passed on to children and grandchildren. This followed on from research done by psychiatrists who suggested practitioners should take a psycho-historical approach to diagnosis and treatment to explore the effects of the Holocaust on third-generation patients. The evidence was suggestive that trauma was biological (Rosenthal and Rosenthal 1980).

There were other examples. Brought up as a Christian, the Canadian author, Alison Pick, said she became profoundly aware of her family's heritage:

> I came to understand it on a bodily level, deep in my cells below my rational mind. I suffer from depression. My family had repressed the horror of the gas chambers. The unfelt grief had been passed from my grandmother to my father to me, like an heirloom. (Pick 2015)

When her relatives migrated to Canada, they hid their Jewish origins. She says of her emotional state: 'the depression I suffer from has always felt pre-formed, ancient, like it was given to me in its entirety at birth.' In her case, trauma came through from generations beyond the grave (Pick 2015).

This topic was addressed by other authors who had memories of the past, a past beyond their birth which appeared to come from someone else's existence. One example of Holocaust memories was included in the novel by Yael Shahar (2014), another by the psychotherapist Elise Wardle (2014) and by Rabbi Gershom (1992) who also wrote on the Holocaust and reincarnation.

One final story was reported second-hand, but with interesting details. This story was published by Trutz Hardo (2005), and he wrote about the visionary Professor Eli Lasch, who fled from Germany to Palestine in 1936. Lasch claimed to have witnessed a three-year-old Druze boy in the Golan Heights who remembered a past life. Druze people had their own religion, of which reincarnation was a part: they believed they would always reincarnate as Druze.

The boy claimed he had been murdered four years earlier and took the elders to a village where he pointed out the murderer who confessed to the crime. Then he took village elders to the place where he said his body was buried and where the axe that killed him was hidden.

CULTURAL PERSPECTIVES ON MENTAL WELLBEING

The skull of the body had an axe wound and the three-year-old boy had a birthmark in the same place.

IMPLICATIONS OF SURVIVAL BELIEFS

What are the implications of survival beliefs? I have wondered whether the beliefs are veridical or hallucinatory. The psychiatrist Viktor Frankl (2008) survived a Nazi concentration camp and he has suggested meaning in life was more important for humans' survival than happiness. His experiences in the camp led him to try and find the most important aspect to human existence. He discovered meaningfulness was key to a person's survival in dire circumstances (Esfahani Smith 2014).

I mention Frankl because he actually survived Auschwitz, whereas the data above suggested other people like Shahar, Wardle and Pick appeared to have had Holocaust memories but were not there personally. I am interested in the Holocaust as I too have had memories which appeared to come from beyond birth, but which were not epigenetic.

I wondered if there were others who had done similar research with those who had memories but who were not descended directly from survivors of the Holocaust. Who has conducted research on the effects of seemingly past life memories on pre-natal emotional development apart from Ian Stevenson's physical influences suggestive of reincarnation?

Was it possible that these other elements and 'memories' might also influence people who have 'mental health' episodes? Was it possible that some of these 'memories' went beyond the effects of childhood and trauma in their present life and beyond their parents' memories of trauma; perhaps they crept into memories of distant incarnations?

Research has suggested that children with memories of past lives also suffered from PTSD. This was a different explanatory model for PTSD. 'Children who report memories of violent deaths in past lives may suffer from post-traumatic stress disorder (PTSD), according to psychologist Dr Erlendur Haraldsson, professor emeritus at the University of Iceland in Reykjavik' (MacIsaac 2014a). Haraldsson offered data to suggest reincarnation was a reality (2012).

If this was true, were those who had mental distress, spiritual awakenings or extreme experiences responding not only to trauma from their current incarnation but also from a previous incarnation?

» 136 «

Or were they tuning in sensitively to a current or earlier scenario? Is it possible to have PTSD from a remote memory? Writing about suicide in Northern Ireland for the Wellcome Trust, the journalist Lyra McKee (2016) has suggested that the 'problems faced in a war-torn country do not end with the arrival of peace'.

PTSD is not new. The military psychologist Professor Hacker Hughes and his team at Anglia Ruskin University have analyzed translations from ancient Mesopotamia from 1300BCE. They say that soldiers gave accounts of being visited by 'ghosts they faced in battle' which is similar to the testimonies of today's soldiers and would fit with the contemporary diagnosis of PTSD (Gallagher 2015). The condition as an effect of warfare could be as old as human civilization itself.

The material above makes me question the 'diseases of the brain' model of mental ill health. It seems that actual or recalled trauma is a trigger of distress. This illustrates the need for patients to be invited to recount their narratives of deep history.

Jamie Horder has questioned the popular 'fact' that one in four people experiences mental ill health and he has suggested this just reinforces our assumptions (2010). It appeared that anyone could experience mental ill health depending on their life circumstances and history. Even the Director-General of the World Health Organization linked mental health to brain disorders – but was she correct to do so? 'Mental illness is not a personal failure. In fact, if there is failure, it is to be found in the way we have responded to people with mental and brain disorders' (WHO 2001). In order to respond better to people who have suffered, is it perhaps time for a cultural U-turn in terms of these statistics and this kind of mindset about diagnosis and treatment?

SUMMARY

Rachel Carson, an American marine biologist, was very interested in the environment. As a writer she said: 'There is something infinitely healing in the repeated refrains of nature, the assurance that dawn comes night after night, and spring after winter' (1999, p.279). Why would nature have a cycle of activity, life and death, whilst human beings do not? The texts above illustrate that many people in many countries believe in survival beyond death. Is this superstition or do they have access to a veridical spiritual reality?

Ethnographic literature suggests people's beliefs about dying and survival beyond death influence their interpretation of mental health symptoms. This chapter was written to explore cultural beliefs about what happened after death and the implications for those who remain; it also explored a wide variety of cultural frameworks and beliefs about survival beyond death. It has presented knowledge from different societies and has looked at reincarnation beliefs in several countries, suggesting that Hindu Indian societies were not the only peoples to hold such thoughts.

The philosophies of the Swiss psychiatrist Elizabeth Kübler-Ross about the time of dying and those of the Indian seer and philosopher Sri Aurobindo were mentioned. As well as exploring death rituals from India, and relatives' intentions to ensure the safety of their ancestors, I also considered concepts like reincarnation and bereavement returnees.

I presented western beliefs about survival beyond death, based on evidence from Ian Stevenson which was suggestive of reincarnation, and from the GP Dewi Rees who suggested it was normal for bereaved people to experience a presence or vision of their deceased partners.

In each faith there may be a variety of beliefs about death and dying and not one clear statement – for example, some Christians and Jews may believe that there is absolute death at the end of life, whereas those Jews who follow the Kabbalah believe in an afterlife, and likewise those Christians who hold spiritist beliefs. I covered the difficult topic of intergenerational ancestral memories and the research that is currently underway exploring this.

Where does this material leave us? In the next few chapters I will consider our dilemma regarding extreme experiences and consciousness beyond the body. I will explore religious experiences in more detail, near-death experiences, cultural interpretation of experiences and spiritual awakening.

Today, groups are emerging who want their anomalous experiences to be interpreted and treated in more compassionate, spiritual ways. A recent book on psychiatry by Whitaker and Cosgrove (2015) makes it feel as if a turning point has been reached.The evidence is there, and we cannot turn away from it. We can no longer deny it. There can be no going back. Issues illustrating the dilemmas of interpretation and consensus about what is or is not 'correct' human experience follows.

10

ANOMALOUS EXPERIENCES

A. Religious and Spiritual Experiences

The American artist, Paige Bradley, created a very moving statue:
a bronze sculpture of a woman seeking inner peace, with her body
fractured open by light. The woman appeared to be a container
for spiritual search, and a powerful voice for healing.

OVERVIEW

In the previous chapter, I mentioned that a turning point has been reached in psychiatry and in the interpretation of anomalous experiences. In this and the following chapters I will explore what Alister Hardy and Seyyed Hossein Nasr thought about religious experiences and the deeper existential realities of being human.

The English biologist, Sir Alister Hardy, commented on our need to know more about religious experiences:

> for years anthropologists have been collecting accounts of religious attitudes, ideas, and feelings from primitive peoples. As a result we know much more about the religious feelings of Polynesians, North American Indians, and various tribes in Africa than we do about those of our fellow citizens in Western society. (1997, p6)

When he retired in 1969, he established the Religious Experience Research Centre which today holds over 6000 narratives of people's experiences. Today it has changed its name to the Alister Hardy Society for the Study of Spiritual Experience (AHSSSE).

Similarly, the American Islamic philosopher Professor Seyyed Hossein Nasr has claimed that society appeared to know a lot about the functioning of the human body, but that we were not aware of the deeper realities of being human. 'The scientific study of the human body has taught mankind a great detail about its functioning but has also veiled much of its reality'. He continued: 'one observes everywhere the attempt to rediscover the deeper significance of the human body, of this bridge to the world of enchanted nature and link to our inner being from which modern man became alienated through the same process that alienated him from the external world of nature' (Nasr 1996, p.256).

This chapter considers spontaneous religious and spiritual experiences, as does the following Chapter 11 on near-death and out-of-body experiences. I present material from two of my research projects on the topic. Chapter 12 discusses the phenomenology of mental health events or extreme experiences, while Chapter 13 presents specialists who deliberately shift consciousness.

The aim is to explore whether there might be any parallels between mental wellbeing, spiritual awakening and anomalous experiences. I look at what people believe about existential realities and the kinds of experiences that human beings have. I explore those human experiences which are believed to be on a continuum from normal to anomalous to abnormal, including the assumed symptoms of 'mental ill health' and spiritual emergency.

I will present a range of meanings our society/civilization gives to the term spirituality and the relevance of such for medicine and healthcare. The following topics are covered in this chapter: unusual human experiences; definition of normal experiences; interdimensional specialists; and the nature of being human.

UNUSUAL HUMAN EXPERIENCES
Historical examples

Throughout history, people have recorded their religious experiences which have often been respected by those who had them and by those people around them. For example, three thousand years ago, Moses saw the Angel of God in a burning bush and he was given a strategy to help his people out of oppression. In 1837, Florence Nightingale heard the voice of God telling her to set up hospitals for the sick; she listened and created our first health service.

In 1858 the visionary Bernadette Soubirous saw the Virgin Mary at Lourdes, at a place which is now a centre of pilgrimage and healing for sick people. Lourdes is a small market town in the foothills of the Pyrenees in south-western France. Today the sanctuary of Our Lady of Lourdes is a place of mass pilgrimage from Europe and other parts of world. Spring water from the grotto is believed to possess healing properties, and around 200 million people have visited the shrine since 1860. The Roman Catholic Church officially recognized 69 healings as 'miraculous', the most recent in July 2013. The healing at Lourdes 'remains unexplained according to current scientific knowledge'.

There was one unusual case recorded in 1984 and published by a psychiatrist in the *British Medical Journal*. In this case a London woman told her doctor that hallucinatory voices in her head were telling her to have a brain scan. He referred her immediately to a psychiatrist. The voice said: 'Please don't be afraid. I know it must be shocking for you to hear me speaking to you like this, but this is the easiest way I could think of. My friend and I used to work at the Children's Hospital, Great Ormond Street, and we would like to help you' (Azuonye 1997, p.1685).

The psychiatrist referred her for a scan, but that department refused, saying she was mentally ill. As the voices became more persistent, the psychiatrist demanded she have a scan to put her mind at rest. The brain scan found she had a tumour which was operated on immediately. After the operation, the voices told her: 'we are pleased to have helped you. Goodbye.' The psychiatrist Dr Azuonye (1997) presented various biomedical and psychological explanations for the appearance and disappearance of her voices. How can we explain these occurrences?

Religious and spiritual experiences

There are a number of different interpretations of the term 'religious experience'. It seems to be a catch-all term with a range of significances. Furthermore, the people who have had experiences can come from any section of the population and they can be of any age, any faith and any ethnic group.

Marianne Rankin's book currently provides the most comprehensive information on the topic (2005). She notes that experiences may have religious, mystical, spiritual, numinous, paranormal or clairvoyant aspects. Transformational religious experiences differ from ordinary experiences. People may experience a kind of non-sensory apprehension of the divine which may manifest itself as transcendence, the numinous or as a higher power. The experiences may or may not be benign. The term also covers people's experience of extended perception, a wider reality, a reality beyond the ordinary or contact with angels or deceased relatives. The topic raises questions about the existence of consciousness beyond death and paranormal experiences.

Altered states of consciousness that specialists deliberately invoke, for example through the consumption of pharmacological substances, trance dancing, focused intention or shamanic drumming are considered later in Chapter 14.

Two research projects into religious experiences

BRUNEL UNIVERSITY

In order to explore anomalous experiences further, I conducted a research project as part of a medical anthropology dissertation for Brunel University (Tobert 2000). The aim was to explore mystical, spiritual and religious experiences. In particular I wanted to examine the polarity between mental health and spiritual experience. The project analyzed respondents' recalled memories of 'religious experiences', initially through a questionnaire and then through selected interviews. I had not specified what I meant by religious experiences as I wanted to explore the respondents' interpretations of that term.

Figure 10.1 sets out the responses to the question as to whether they ever had spontaneous mystical, spiritual or religious experiences. Among respondents, there seemed to be an assumption that negative experiences were an indication of mental ill health. This needed exploring further.

HAVE YOU EVER HAD MYSTICAL, SPIRITUAL OR RELIGIOUS EXPERIENCE(S) BY CHANCE?

Out of 60 questionnaire and interview responses, 45 people replied in the affirmative.

Types of experiences:

- transcendental: connection with nature / universe – 7 11%
- experiences of love, light, and God – 8 13%
- body changes, OBE's, *kundalini* (energy) rising – 9 15%
- extra-sensory perception: warnings, clairvoyance – 9 15%
- presences: of angels, or deceased human beings 13 21%

The circumstances

- in nature
- suffering
- sudden trauma
- everyday situations
- whilst using substances
- sleeping, dreaming, or liminal states
- during meditation, yoga, relaxation, or prayer

Effects

- calm, joy, bliss
- disoriented, surprised
- developed different spiritual abilities
- experience provided a life turning point
- changed perception about western thought

Explanatory models

- I can't, I don't need to
- I'm unable to, it's beyond understanding
- God, angels, spirits…were looking after me
- other dimensions, underlying reality to this world
- omnipresent divine energies, the supernatural

Brunel University MSc Project, 2000

Figure 10.1. Mystical Experiences, Brunel University Data

During my survey on religious experiences, I asked whether the respondents had ever been diagnosed as having a mental illness. Nine people answered this question. One woman, traumatized by her mother's attempts at exorcism, was later diagnosed with depression. Another who saw multiple levels of reality simultaneously (including spirits of the dead) was diagnosed with depression, mania and dissociative disorder. She was hospitalized for a brief period and prescribed anti-depressants and tranquillizers. However, she did not think she had a mental health problem, and many years later she heard about neo-shamanic practices, which valued visionary experiences and taught deliberate disassociation and controlled return to common consensus reality. Today she is a businesswoman in the USA.

Alister Hardy Centre

I also conducted a second research project with the Alister Hardy Research Centre. In the 1970s Sir Alister Hardy created an archive of personal narratives from people who claimed to have had a religious experience. He used the media to invite the public to send in their experiences and then conducted systematic studies of the texts. He felt the significance of such a study would throw light on the nature of life itself. It appeared the research he initiated threw light not only on the nature of life, but also on consciousness beyond death and beyond the body.

The archives were kept at the Religious Experience Research Centre at the University of Wales in Lampeter. The aim of my research project was to explore explanatory models for religious experiences perceived as negative or considered as warranting psychiatric assistance. I sampled the database on people's attitudes and observers' assumptions as to whether religious experiences warranted psychiatric attention.

I was interested in the *response* to the experience (by family, friends and religious or medical professionals) rather than the *content*. I wanted to hear about experients' own responses and the responses and attitudes of those personal and professional observers around them. I wanted to know how people explained the experience and how it fitted into their framework of understanding about the nature of human existence.

In those years there had been considerable discussion about whether religious experiences were pathological or not. In theory, this was really clear. Within psychiatry, having religious experiences per se was not indicative of pathology; only by having a combination of symptoms would a person be considered mentally ill. The ability to function in everyday life and not be of harm to oneself or others was critical.

However, the data I uncovered at the Religious Experience Research Centre suggested there was a mismatch between public perception and the most sensitive and aware psychiatrists. I wanted to explore the nature of this mismatch, to determine its extent with regard to religious experiences and its currency over time. I wanted to know to what extent pathology was still proposed as a response to religious experiences.

The research discovered that there was often a stigma or silence attached to having religious experiences. Some people who had them didn't speak about them for fear of being misunderstood or being thought foolish or insane. Respondents said it was 'quite impossible for me to speak of my feelings of experiences, and indeed, I have never done so up to this time' and 'I never speak of these things I have told you' and 'One never spoke of such things' (Tobert 2007, p.41). There was a link between the fear of insanity and speaking out. There was an underlying assumption (among some respondents) that a visionary religious experience was a symptom of mental illness, of schizophrenia. I found out that a mismatch existed between popular and professional perceptions of religious experiences.

Popular misperceptions existed in spite of professional reassurances from psychiatrists. Respondents convinced themselves they were having dreams. As one person who saw an angel with wings in a white light explained: 'it then vanished and I awoke, assuming as I do for the sake of my sanity that it was a dream'. Another said 'doctors laughed at my fears of impending insanity but I forced an interview with a psychiatrist. He offered nothing except that I was an interesting case' (Tobert 2007, p.44).

Some experients did have contact with a psychiatrist, although other respondents were unwilling to accept the label of psychosis after having had an experience. Others were grateful for the psychiatric treatment they received. Some underwent extensive medical tests to determine the pathology that caused the experience. In order to understand their experience, some spoke to religious and medical professionals and seemed disappointed at their response. One man who experienced the voice of god directly said: 'my psychiatrist, a wonderful man, relies on shock treatment and pills to control it [the voice]' (Tobert 2007, p.47).

In the 1970s, a woman saw a brilliant white light come through the top of her head. She went to several doctors, had her eyes examined, had an ECG, x-rays for a brain tumour and visited a psychiatrist. 'None of them could find anything physically or mentally wrong with me'. She continued: 'Feeling desperately lonely because I had no one to share my experience, I sought out a psychiatrist to see if I could communicate with someone, but he had no idea what I was talking about. I asked the Chaplain and he ignored me' (Tobert 2007, p.49).

There appeared to be a fine line between psychosis and spirituality. Respondents thought religious or spiritual experiences and psychosis existed within a continuum. In the 1980s archive staff noted that it was difficult to tell the difference between symptoms of schizophrenia and religious experiences. In spite of the ideal level of awareness about spirituality and psychosis, in actual practice there seemed to be a gap at frontline healthcare services for experients.

People had different responses to the experiences. One said, 'religious experience, paranormal experience, the experience of insanity and also the inspiration of genius, may all spring from the same source'. Another claimed that 'the dividing line between insanity and revelation involving high spiritual perception is very fine indeed'. Another person commented that 'the phenomenon is so traumatic that most patients come to accept the diagnosis of the psychiatrists, rather than face up to the memory of what they actually experienced themselves' (Tobert 2007, p.56).

It became obvious during the research project that religious practice and religious experiences were given different values by society: religious practice was ubiquitously considered a virtue, whereas religious experience was feared, misunderstood or pathologized.

What exactly is our self?

Alister Hardy collected data which could be used to inform studies of consciousness, survival after death and paranormal events (1997). Research data from my two research projects illustrated that respondents' narratives suggested the self was experienced in various ways: the boundaries of the self may be fluid; perception may be experienced beyond the body; and, the self may be made up of pre-natal and extra-corporeal experiences as well as post-natal psychological responses.

Our ways of understanding religious experience changed over time and our concept of 'normal' evolved. Pathological symptoms of mental illness were clearly defined, but in terms of religious or 'anomalous' experiences, research suggested that different people interpreted the same symptoms in different ways, and different professions addressed similar symptoms in different ways.

In the past, professionals tended to pathologize experiences that they didn't understand or that didn't fit within a materialist paradigm. Over time, our beliefs have changed and our responses to religious experiences have been modified and adapted. To what extent do our beliefs about the nature of reality still influence our understanding and interpretation of anomalous experiences?

SUMMARY

This chapter has presented the results of two research projects. I have provided examples of visionary religious experiences which have been accepted over time, including that of Moses, Florence Nightingale and the Virgin Mary at Lourdes.

My intention has been to have scholars who study anomalous and paranormal experiences to consider carefully the phenomena and compare them to those of people diagnosed with mental health problems. It seemed that the vocabulary around experiences could be interpreted in several ways, depending on the belief system of the observer.

In the next chapter I also consider people who have had spontaneous near death or out of body experiences, but these have been studied in great detail in their own right, and so have been mentioned separately.

11

ANOMALOUS EXPERIENCES

B. Near-Death Experiences (NDE), Out-of-Body Experiences (OBE), End-of-Life Experiences (ELE)

OVERVIEW

There are other kinds of human experiences which used to come under the umbrella of religious experiences but which are now studied in their own right. They have attracted a wealth of literature, in particular by the International Association for Near-Death Studies. In this chapter I will address experiences which occur spontaneously and stop. These unusual human experiences may occur within healthcare settings and have attracted the attention of psychiatrists, cardiologists and those working in intensive care units.

The intention is to discuss the relevance of near-death and out-of-body experiences for healthcare practice and mental health in particular. I will present spontaneous experiences that occur to human beings, without their having taken any action to invoke them. These include: religious experiences; near-death experiences and out-of-body experiences.

Deliberate action taken by people in order to have an experience is addressed in Chapter 14. The text below is not intended as an in-depth presentation of the material as that can be found elsewhere. It is simply a snapshot. My proposal is that some people who spontaneously have these experiences may not have a framework for understanding them, and, in association with other factors, they may attract psychiatric attention.

These experiences matter because in the past they may have been interpreted ad hoc, depending on the belief system of the observer or beholder (Tobert 2007, Betty 2009). In some cases experients were pathologized.

Although in theory it is clear what is and is not a mental health problem, in practice, in the past, the boundaries were muddied, for example when people could not stop the experience at will and when both they and those around them did not have relevant frameworks for understanding. This is why this book has been written – to offer new frameworks for understanding and interpreting experiences and, in the long term, to reduce the distress of experients.

In earlier times, having visionary or auditory experiences was often taken as an indicator of mental ill health, but these days this occurs less frequently. During research with the Alister Hardy Society Archive, I found that negative experiences were assumed to be indicative of 'mental illness' whereas positive ones were assumed to be 'religious' (Tobert 2007).

In a paper accompanying the Alister Hardy report, I explored what our beliefs were about being human and the kinds of experiences we consider it normal to have. In the past people were hesitant about making a link between religious experiences, but today this is often discussed. The *Journal of Religious and Spiritual Experiences* is now available online at the University of Wales.

NEAR-DEATH EXPERIENCES
Near-death and anomalous experiences

The oldest medical description of the phenomenon of NDE may come from a French physician in around 1740. It scored 12 points on the Greyson scale which measures NDE. This was seen in a report written by Pierre-Jean du Monchaux (1776). The psychologist Stanley Krippner has talked about the transformational aspects of spiritual experiences and he has explained why professionals should know about them (2012). Furthermore, the International Association for Near-Death Studies has suggested that healthcare workers should not treat people who have near-death experiences as mentally ill (MacIsaac 2014b).

The London neuro-psychiatrist, Peter Fenwick, was renowned for his research into NDE and end-of-life phenomena (Fenwick and Fenwick 1995). He conducted an investigation of over 300 NDEs, illustrating the narratives of hospital patients who appeared to leave their body and view it from above. They travelled through tunnels and saw a bright light. A few travelled outside the room (undertaking remote viewing) and saw situations occurring elsewhere, although very few travelled any great distance. They reported seeing deceased or religious figures, visions of the future, brilliant lights and they felt as though they had extrasensory perception.

For a period, near-death experiences became a catch-all term for any kind of experience, even though the experient was not near death but they reported similar phenomena.

Some were defined as out-of-body experiences. There was one example from the UK. I heard about it when I attended a talk given by Dr Joan LaRovere who was Associate Director of Paediatric Intensive Care at the Royal Brompton Hospital in London. She reported on a journey she took as she escorted a fourteen-year-old child to another hospital in an ambulance.

She explained that the child had a brain tumour and had suffered cardiac arrest several times before being transferred. On the journey, as the child arrested again, the vehicle stopped and the crew tried resuscitation. Dr LaRovere realized the girl was clinically dead but insisted the ambulance continue to its end destination, since she knew the child's parents would be waiting.

A row broke out: ambulance crews are supposed to convey the deceased to the nearest hospital. Tempers were frayed, a telephone was dropped and chaos ensued. Eventually, the patient was revived. A year later, when Dr LaRovere asked what the patient recalled about her time in the hospital, the child remembered the ambulance ride well and all the fluster. The doctor was shocked because the girl had been clinically dead throughout the ride. This was her first experience of hearing about non-corporeal consciousness.

Among French speakers, the *Manuel clinique des expériences extraordinaires* (*The Clinical Handbook of Extraordinary Experiences*) represented a collaborative project between many writers about their insights into extraordinary experiences (Allix and Bernstein 2009). The authors suggested a clinical approach that was suitable for healthcare providers to better understanding the experiences. They suggested that the greatest risk to someone who has had experiences was when those around them pathologized them: they advised that it was better to suspend judgement.

The manual presented chapters on near-death experiences and end-of-life experiences by my colleague Evelyn Elsaesser-Valarino (2001). She has written numerous books on NDE and has worked closely with Kenneth Ring, an American professor of psychology. One of his most memorable stories was a narrative gathered about unusual experiences from a woman who had been blind since birth (2008).

BELIEFS ABOUT CONSCIOUSNESS BEYOND LIFE

Pim van Lommel, a Dutch cardiologist who has studied NDEs in patients who survived cardiac arrest, published a study on NDEs in *The Lancet* (2001). He claimed our beliefs about the relationship between the brain and consciousness was too narrow to be able to understand the phenomenon. He gave examples of ways that consciousness does not always coincide with brain function and could be experienced separately from the body. His new book contains robust evidence that consciousness continued after the death of the body (van Lommel 2011).

OBEs

The American psychologist, Charles Tart (1997), has clearly defined an OBE and has explained that the main characteristic of it was the feeling that a person's centre of perception was located somewhere outside the body. Although the person's eyes were physically still in their head, the person's perception was above, beyond or outside their body. In an OBE the mind was clearly separate from the body, although it was capable of the same level of rational thought.

Spontaneous out-of-body experiences may occur to anyone in any place and there have been many reports of them occurring in healthcare settings. I will present data and narratives collected from within medical or healthcare settings. These are interesting because patients' comments are linked to the procedure and medical records.

MICHAEL SABOM AND PAM REYNOLDS

In America in the 1990s, the cardiovascular physician Michael Sabom (1998) started to conduct research into out-of-body experiences in hospital. He was particularly interested in their relation to religion and Christianity. One of the best documented case studies was in 1991: a woman called Pam Reynolds had close medical monitoring during an entire operation for brain surgery.

Pam, a 35-year-old woman, described the procedures which she perceived during an operation for an aneurysm. Sabom informed us that her body temperature was lowered to 60 degrees: her heartbeat and breathing stopped; her brainwaves flattened and the blood was drained from her head. She was temporarily dead with no measurable brain function.

Pam Reynolds was a professional musician and she told doctors the drill which opened up her skull vibrated like a D natural. This instrument had not been used until she was totally unconscious and none of the doctors had a clue about the musical note at which the drill vibrated, but she was right. She saw the operating room from above, watched them shave her head and described the tools they used for bone surgery.

She could also hear the medical team's conversation as the operation progressed. She said 'it was the most aware I think I have ever been in my entire life'...'it was not like normal vision. It was brighter and more focused and clearer than normal vision.' (Sabom 1998) She saw a tunnel, heard her grandmother's voice, saw many of her family members who had died and she perceived a bright light. This was one of the most renowned cases, as there was full medical documentation of her operation which was correlated to the timings presented in her comments.

Non-corporeal vision

Kenneth Ring was a professor of psychology at Connecticut University when he became interested in near-death experiences and non-corporeal vision. One of the more significant case studies was an interview with Vicki Umipeg who found herself floating above her body in the emergency room of a hospital following a car accident. She was aware of being up near the ceiling watching a male doctor and a female nurse working on her body which she viewed from her elevated position.

Then she travelled up through the ceilings of the hospital until she was *above* the roof of the building itself, during which time she had a brief panoramic view of her surroundings. She felt very exhilarated and said she began to hear sublimely harmonious music. Her case was unusual because of her extraocular vision: she was congenitally blind, her optic nerve having been destroyed at birth (Ring 2008).

Science and OBEs

Sam Parnia, a cardiologist, and other scientists at Southampton University claimed to have found evidence that awareness continued for a few moments after clinical death (2007). He also oversaw a large study of 2,000 people who had a heart attack and recovered, with a cohort from 15 hospitals in the United Kingdom, the United States and Austria (Parnia *et al.* 2014).

The study used rigorous methods to ensure the data would be of scientific interest. They wanted to record any cognitive experiences that occurred during cardiac arrest. The data suggested 40% of people who survived a cardiac arrest were aware that they were clinically dead before their hearts restarted.

Parnia participated in an event at Imperial College, London with Horizon Research, where scientists collaborated in discussions about consciousness, the soul and the self. He was a medical emergency doctor who became very interested in consciousness beyond the brain and he suggested how we might change our expectations about death and resuscitation.

End-of-life experiences (ELE)

Near-death experiences were a catch-all term for experiences that people had whether or not they were near death, whereas end-of-life experiences were a phenomenon particular to dying people. The term came into popular usage early in the twenty-first century. The psychiatrist Peter Fenwick conducted research into deathbed phenomena and into end-of-life experiences and their impact on relatives and friends. Together with Sue Brayne, he conducted a five-year retrospective study into end-of-life experiences (2011).

They discovered that sometimes those dying wanted to talk about and acknowledge the process of dying. The consensus among certain scholars was that at the end of life, the line between mundane reality and a person's inner space narrowed. It became thin. Some dying people claimed to be visited by pre-deceased relatives or pets, or even religious figures that came to support them on their next journey.

People dying may have a life review, whilst others may stare fixedly at something the observer cannot witness. Peter Fenwick suggested some people visited relatives remotely, in other rooms or other countries.

How should we respond to this? By suggesting they are confused, delusional or that their experiences are veridical? This depends on our own (subjective) belief system.

Fenwick and his colleagues suggested we should listen carefully without prejudice to the experiences of the dying and engage with them with gentle touching and prayers if appropriate. Figure 11.1 gives a series of suggestions that were generated during an interview with Peter Fenwick by Iain McNay in 2012.

- 10 percent of people who have cardiac arrest have a near death experience.
- Many people will have a premonition that they are going to die within two days before.
- Or, they will be visited by a dead relative.
- Death-bed visions are the next step. This prepares the person who is going to die for death.
- Common visions: relatives and spiritual figures tell the dying person that they will be back to pick them up. Sometimes they even tell the dying person the date that they will die.
- The dying person can negotiate the postponement of their death by a little. For example, the dying person can ask for a postponement until after a close friend or relative arrives.
- The next thing that happens for some that are dying is that they go into another reality and come back. They go to an area that is full of love, light, spiritual beings and relatives. It's very much like a near-death experience.
- Paralyzed people are sometimes able to sit up and Alzheimer's patients sometime regain their memory for periods of time just before death.
- The dying person will sometimes visit someone they are emotionally attached to. Space and time are no factor.
- The dying person sees a mirage, sparks and radiant light.
- As far as dying is concerned, clearly consciousness is something special in the way that consciousness fragments and leaves the body.

Advice: if you can, be with your loved ones when they die. Take your cues from them.

Figure 11.1. McNay interview with Dr Peter Fenwick

Penny Sartori, who was an intensive care nurse at a Welsh hospital, made a deep connection with a dying patient early in her career. This initiated her research into near-death experiences (2008). She realized death-bed visions were common and had been under-reported as people struggled to interpret their experiences. A website has now been set up to signpost people to peer support and help them through these transformational experiences.[1]

SUMMARY

My suggestion in this chapter has been that some people who have suffered from extreme experiences may be experiencing an NDE, OBE or ELE. In the past, they may have attracted psychiatric attention.

I was interested in the relevance of these phenomena in terms of the experiences had by people who have been pathologized and described as having a mental health condition. My intention was to explore whether there are any similarities between such phenomena and extreme or anomalous experiences.

If we didn't pathologize visionary or auditory experiences, would we develop different diagnostic and treatment strategies for people having extreme experiences? I will explore this in Chapter 13 and will present new treatment practices in Chapter 16.

In the next chapter I will look at cultural interpretations of anomalous experiences. By cultural in this context I mean people who might be non-white or non-Christian (although the term 'cultural' becomes difficult in intercity areas of the UK and the USA, which flourish with heterogeneous complexity). I already mentioned my problem with the term 'white' in Chapter 2. From a political perspective, it feels as if today's society is treated as if it were homogeneous, with our governments having no need to be aware of different people's beliefs around health and life. The following chapter will explore this.

---

1   www.neardeathexperienceuk.com

12

ANOMALOUS EXPERIENCES

C. Cultural Interpretations of Mental Health

INTRODUCTION

Of all the topics covered in this book, the question as to what is or isn't a mental health problem is possibly the most contentious. This chapter covers the different ways people interpret their symptoms or their conditions (it has been said that the word 'symptom' in itself is value laden). I will look at the assumptions around the terms 'knowledge' and 'belief' and will suggest that agreed consensus at a particular time usually determines what is correct or true.

I will give an example of a mental health promotion project that focused on different religions which I facilitated in a London borough. This has been included to stress the importance of using multiple frameworks for addressing mental wellbeing. I also mention the research I carried out in India on religion, spirituality and mental health.

I live and work in the London Borough of Harrow where, according to the council's Vitality Profiles (2011–13), one-third of residents were born abroad, in 137 different countries, including Iran, Afghanistan, Eastern European countries, Somalia and the countries of the Middle East. The population born outside UK (first-generation migrants) often have different health needs from those born in the UK.

We need to consider a plurality of perspectives when offering healthcare to people of different ethnicities. One size does not fit all. Difficulties may arise if patient and practitioner beliefs about the causes of ill health are in conflict. This may occur particularly when dealing with first generation migrants. They may not trust the diagnosis or refuse the treatment unless the practitioner has made appropriate efforts to communicate with them, both to hear and acknowledge their explanatory models and negotiate an agreed treatment solution.

In Chapter 7 I considered some of the topics here and presented ways in which consensus and public opinion have changed on issues that were assumed to be indicative of mental illness. I presented a series of cultural U-turns in terms of mental health and society: this included having a child outside of marriage; being a child born out of wedlock; being gay or lesbian or the acknowledgement of the triggers of mental distress.

I noted earlier that there were plural cultural frameworks of belief, knowledge and understanding. In the past there seemed to be an 'us and them' approach: i.e. we (westerners) had 'knowledge' whereas the others had 'beliefs'. In particular I discussed the relevance of religious and spirituality experiences for the mental wellbeing of BAME migrants and refugee populations.

People's beliefs about their experiences influence their explanatory models for certain symptoms of distress and may affect their access to healthcare and compliance with treatment. There is a need for cultural humility – to ask the right questions during a consultation.

WESTERN CULTURAL BELIEFS
Host populations

Let us grasp the nettle of culture and ethnicity. In certain areas of the UK, the term 'western culture' is not meaningful. I don't know what it means to me. It doesn't mean white, it doesn't mean Anglo-Saxon and it doesn't mean Christian. I don't think it means capitalist or democratic. When I talk about the populations of some London boroughs where the so-called ethnic minority populations are the majority, then western culture is a rich mix of heterogeneous influences. In some towns the host population is a dynamic ethnic mix but at what point and after how many years do migrants become considered as the 'host population'? At what point do we become fully enculturated? Perhaps I mean Eurocentric beliefs?

In order to discern cultural influences around mental health, I might use the terms biomedical beliefs, or reductionist beliefs, compared to spiritual or religious beliefs, or beliefs of people who are new migrants. During 2007 the government was already aware that BME groups were over-represented in the mental health system.

The Count Me In census had raised awareness that African people were more likely to be sectioned (44%) under the Mental Health Act (CQC 2011, p.3) and the topic of institutional racism was raised. I have not grasped the nettle of ethnicity and inequalities here, but others like Suman Fernando (2014), Bhui and Bhugra (2002b) and Vige *et al.* (2009) have addressed the complexities in detail.

London, UK. Clinical healthcare staff

Beliefs are important because they may influence a person's access to medical and healthcare services. I undertook a Needs Assessment (Tobert 2008) and then facilitated a programme of mental health promotion with different cultural and religious groups in North West London. It was entitled Bridging Cultures, Dissolving Barriers (Tobert 2010a).

The aim was to address inequalities in access to mental health services with Harrow's BAME communities (and refugee and asylum seekers) and to raise awareness about the cultural and religious understandings of mental health with medical and healthcare staff. Part of my role was to invite psychiatric staff and religious leaders into a room together to explore common understandings of symptoms.

During one BAME mental health promotion exercise with the Crisis Resolution Team at a hospital in North West London, staff were asked about their own beliefs about the end of life. During the ensuing discussions, participants realized their own colleagues, with whom they worked side by side practising clinical care, had quite different understandings about human existence, mental health, life and death. Their training in healthcare was the same or similar but their existential beliefs were often quite different because they came from many different religious faiths. As a result of the project, staff acquired a raised awareness of cultural theories of illness causation: they said the seminar 'helped us consider cultural differences when working with patients'. In that hospital in North West London, the staff participants' countries of origin were Nigeria, Kenya, Mauritius, Zimbabwe, Greece, the UK and Australia and the religions were Catholic, Church of England, Hindu, Muslim and atheist.

This mental health promotion project seemed successful. It was evidence based, seminars were participatory, it was an experiential forum for peer learning and mostly because service users, carers and mental health professionals discussed topics together in the same room. Participants' insights and input created dynamic discussions on beliefs about culture, religion and mental wellbeing and the project acknowledged the important role of religion and faith. We discovered it was important to be aware of our own existential beliefs.

USA, Yale University clinicians' beliefs

An example of research from Yale University illustrates why it is so important for us to reflect on our own paradigms and beliefs. Yale conducted an investigation into mental health clinicians' ontological beliefs about mental disorders (Woo-kyoung *et al.* 2009). Clinicians' beliefs about the biological, psychological and environmental bases of disorders were examined. They investigated the consequences of beliefs for judging the effectiveness of treatment. Researchers found that clinicians treated conditions differently: their beliefs had implications for the effectiveness of psychotherapy or medication and therefore their choice of treatment options for patients was affected. This example illustrates why it is necessary for us to be self-reflexive.

PERSONAL NARRATIVES

This section explores different theories of illness causation and the ways our beliefs influence access to services, the acceptance of diagnosis and treatment. We will look at a range of communication strategies that could be used to honour our own beliefs and engage with the beliefs of clients. Passages here provide a forum for reflective discussion of the relevance of communication for health and wellbeing.

I will address the topic of communication and faith, because poor communication is a topic often cited by patients in complaints about healthcare professionals. The German Swiss psychiatrist and philosopher Karl Jaspers (1959) has said: 'the ultimate thing in the doctor-patient relationship is existential communication, which goes far beyond any therapy, that is, beyond anything that can be planned or methodically staged'. What more might we do to promote spiritual, moral, social and cultural awareness for the benefit of staff and patients?

At times when I have been teaching in the past, I invited seminar participants to tell their personal narratives in small groups, to describe themselves, their faith and their ancestral history of origin.

Although this exercise made some people feel uncomfortable, it allowed participants to reflect on their own values, beliefs and identity. They found narratives were powerful and immediate. When they were with patients, these stories put illness episodes into context and acknowledged a person's culture and faith. They heard real stories from real people and found this the purpose of listening to patient narratives.

The University of Massachusetts Medical School also discovered storytelling was a powerful tool for health promotion in vulnerable populations. They conducted a randomized, controlled trial with 230 African Americans. Their conclusion was that the storytelling intervention produced substantial and significant improvements in blood pressure for patients with baseline uncontrolled hypertension: 'Telling and listening to stories is the way we make sense of our lives' (Houston *et al.* 2011, p.77).

Personal narratives are an excellent strategy to engage with new migrant communities to find out about cultural interpretations of symptoms and people's spiritual and religious beliefs. The underlying assumption here is that people have different ways of understanding human existence and reality in the world. There are many frameworks of understanding.

Ways of understanding health, illness and disease are part of belief systems which may vary with each ethnic group and each religion. Cultural values mean certain individuals within communities may delay consultation with mainstream mental health services. Modern health service provision needs to take account of different cultural beliefs in order to be culturally sensitive and not limit the access of ethnic minorities. The most appropriate and effective mental health promotion projects are ones which both raise awareness of pathways to access healthcare for vulnerable groups and raise staff awareness of cultural beliefs and the need for cultural humility.

In the past, sometimes mental health provision was a one-way service. Carpenter and Raj have suggested there was 'a grudging recognition that mental health services have too often acted in oppressive ways, particularly to groups facing other forms of discrimination on the basis of gender, "race", religion, age, ethnicity and sexuality' (2012, p.457). They wrote that there was renewed hope: 'provided by widespread acceptance of the "recovery" model that emerged from the mental health survivors' movement, challenging the negative tendencies of existing psychiatric services, as well as the discriminatory barriers that need to be overcome in the wider society' (Carpenter and Raj 2012, p.457).

EXPLANATORY MODELS FOR MENTAL DISTRESS

We will consider the topics of migration, mental health diagnosis and religion together: people who are forced into migration from their country of origin or from the place where their ancestors are buried may be more at risk of experiencing episodes of stress, anxiety or mental ill health.

Forced migration may be the result of war or trauma or of holding beliefs incompatible with a country's ruling parties which may result in imprisonment. Living away from the support of extended family and friends can increase social isolation. Religious and spiritual practices are important aspects of daily life, especially for first-generation migrants.

Cultural knowledge and belief

Our beliefs are important: they inform the way we interpret our experiences (our theories of illness causation); they influence our health-seeking practices for our mental wellbeing; and, they influence our access to healthcare and our acceptance of diagnosis and treatments. There are different ways that people both interpret their symptoms of distress and select treatment strategies. People's theories of illness causation may be very different and this influences the healing options they choose.

The medical anthropologist, Byron Good (1994), noted that anthropologists in the past used the term 'belief' in a particular way: culture-bound knowledge was assumed to be 'belief' (i.e. erroneous) and has long been used to connote 'mistaken understandings' whereas 'knowledge' was assumed to mean 'correct explanations'. Cultural knowledge was assumed to be 'belief'.

In this section, I will explore cross-cultural explanations for health and existence and examine people's understandings from their own perspectives. 'Emic' is a term from anthropology, meaning an insider perspective, specific to culture, essential for the empathic understanding of a culture. In contrast, the term 'etic' means the external researcher's perspective which is supposedly 'culturally neutral' and useful for cross-cultural comparison. In the past the debate was that etic knowledge was objective and superior to emic knowledge or subjective belief. However, this was itself a cultural assumption: all of us are enculturated into a particular worldview which we assume is 'the truth'.

The beliefs we hold fit within particular paradigms. They inform our theories of education, behaviour, values and society. They influence what we teach, our theories of illness causation and our health-seeking strategies. A paradigm is a set of assumptions, a worldview or opinion about how we understand our existence in the world. Today, the older paradigms around mental health are being questioned, not only from a 'cultural' perspective but also from a new paradigm of understanding.

Somali migrants and mental health promotion

In the UK new populations of migrants and refugees may interpret and diagnose their symptoms in ways unfamiliar to healthcare staff. Belief systems about the meaning of experiences and symptoms may be quite different in different cultures. Members may interpret symptoms as requiring treatment from religious practitioners (church, temple or mosque and so forth) rather than from clinical practitioners. This may delay people requesting help from mental health service practitioners. Therefore, it may be useful for clinical staff to discuss medical and religious health-seeking strategies with patients.

The transcultural psychiatrist, Suman Fernando, has explained more about culture and belief. In African cultures, the non-physical world was inhabited by the spirits of people who had died, people who were alive and those about to be born, animals, plants and objects without biological life. The spiritual and physical worlds were not separate entities. In psychiatry, mystical or trance states were associated with a 'loss of ego control' and were seen as pathological because 'self-control' was considered important in western culture (Fernando 1991).

Fernando has also explored issues of institutional racism: in the USA, he observed that people of African descent, Hispanics and Native Americans were 'overdiagnosed' as schizophrenic. He commented that 'the use of psychiatric diagnoses cross-culturally is problematic. Black British people of African-Caribbean ethnicity are overrepresented among people given the diagnosis schizophrenia/psychosis.

This situation is explicable in terms of cultural misunderstanding coupled with institutional racism' (Fernando 1991).

Claims about schizophrenia

A similar comment about the overdiagnosis of schizophrenia was made in the UK by a Somali advocate in North West London (Tobert 2010b). He claimed that a high proportion (95%) of his 32 Somali clients were diagnosed with schizophrenia. He considered the issue needed to be addressed as it seemed statistically unlikely to be true. He asked: 'why on earth [do] all these people have the same diagnosis?'

He felt service providers did not understand the importance of hearing service users' narratives and historical backgrounds. New migrants often had religious theories of mental illness causation and feared both stigma and 'government' intervention, which discouraged them from approaching healthcare professionals.

London-based Somalis

In 2010, the London borough of Harrow had over 10,000 Somali residents who suffered deprivation and social exclusion and who had unaddressed mental health problems. The aim of the project was to evaluate the effectiveness of Somali advocacy and to explore cultural understandings of western and Somali models of mental health, family and confidentiality, gender and triggers of distress. The advocate explained about different treatment strategies used by the community. In addition to community mental health services, he said that 'we go to mosques, where they read [the] Koran on you. There are special passages, depending [on] what is disturbing you. We can find cure[s] in Koran. There are religious practitioners who read the Koran here in Harrow' (Tobert 2010b).

A carer said of his relative: 'I took him to a Sheikh. He read the Koran over his head.' The advocate explained:

'Here, Somali people would not want to go to mainstream services, because of the stigma, and also they feel disempowered. They would rather consider alternatives from their own communities, going to family members, or religious practitioners. Very few people want to go with [the] mainstream.' (Tobert 2010b, p.vi)

I interviewed one service provider of African origin. He was frustrated about Eurocentric ways of understanding mental health and he emphasized the importance of learning about a culture and not pathologizing symptoms:

> From a Eurocentric perspective, people just don't get it, they just don't understand. It is important because the understanding of culture is what helps people to get better. There are things that happen in African culture, that may not be acceptable in European culture, but it is their way of life, it doesn't translate to a diagnosis of badness. (Tobert 2010b)

A female colleague of West African origin has commented on issues of race, culture and mental health. In an email to me, she wrote:

> There is disquiet amongst our BME community about how we are treated by the mental health system; it oppresses us instead of helping us. Instead of helping, it demonizes us, causing us to have to fight for justice all the time (on top of having to deal with the problems in hand). We do not want to be viewed/ treated as victims, but with the same dignity and respect.

Mental health promotion needs to be considered from the new migrants' perspective to take account of how they interpret symptoms and their consultation models. This may ease or reduce claims of racism and the promotion of Eurocentric practices.

Possessing spirits, Africa

In the UK, the difference in interpreting a person's symptoms of distress was dependent on the cultural or ethnic group or religion of the observer. One colleague explained her African and Western fusion of the interpretation of symptoms and chosen treatment in an email to me:

> As a survivor of mental health illness myself, I was believing that I am possessed by djinn and spirits. Hearing voices and hallucinations were to me voices of people from the dead and djinn talking to me. I sometime thought of myself as holy. Sometimes I thought I am under the spell of black magic and evil eye. I went through all that for years treated by different Community Mental Health Teams. I am finally sane and recovered, not hearing voices any more, working full time.

An advocate from Somalia explained understandings from his community's perspective:

> When a family see one of their relatives mentally ill, straightaway they find a sheikh, who can read specific Qur'anic verses over them, and have the power to heal. This is absolutely different from an imam, who reads prayers in a mosque. The sheikh has special knowledge about djinn, and how to treat them. When Somali people came to Harrow, they didn't change these practices: to them medication is secondary, and they try to avoid taking it.

He also explained the problems of stigma and isolation: 'Because of the stigma of mental illness, people become confined within their families' (Tobert 2010, p.vi). The advocate said that people with symptoms of distress were hidden in their homes, unseen by the mental health services.

The anthropologist Lewis (1969) did fieldwork in Somalia from the 1950s onwards. He explained ubiquitous beliefs in the existence of spirits: certain kinds of illness resulted from a spirit or *djinn* entering a person and making them physically or mentally ill. This could also occur as the result of a curse. However, when a spirit entered a person 'with permission' to give them beneficial information, this was known as mediumship. The treatment the Somalis used for spirit possession was to receive a blessing (*baraka*) from the Koran. The blessing was read over the patient by a sheikh, or written into an amulet, and for women there was a ceremony known as Zar exorcism.

People from Africa and elsewhere may worry because they know that their symptoms, causes and meanings of illness may be rather different from those of western medical and healthcare practitioners. They fear medicine may be used to treat their symptoms rather than the cause of them. Diagnosis may indicate a western 'cause' of ill health but it does not determine the 'meaning' for the client.

Islamic cultural perspectives

I once visited an Islamic bookshop in North West London and saw a notice on the wall; it was an advertisement offering exorcism. I phoned the number and then met the sheikh who offered the service. I asked him what symptoms could result in a diagnosis of spirit possession.

The sheikh told me about Islamic cultural perspectives and gave his explanation of the symptoms people described to him.

Symptoms, he said, included severe headaches (not alleviated by painkillers), mood swings, anxiety, distress, depression, seizures and infertility (that had no medical cause) and the hearing of voices (*waswas* or whispering). In addition to physical ailments, he explained human beings were also susceptible to other influences like witchcraft, the evil eye, destructive envy, spirit possession or *djinn* possession.

His treatment was to recite prayers over the person. He was a specialist reader and not an imam offering prayers in the mosque. He told me about Islamic cultural treatment. According to scholars, there was no contradiction between Islam and the medical sciences. His recommendations for mental ill health were to use Islamic treatments after medical treatment had been exhausted. Patients should consult a qualified medical practitioner at the onset of their symptoms and should continue taking prescribed medication whilst consulting or reciting Islamic texts to help ease symptoms.

Another scholar told me about the writings of the prophet and the ways in which patients might respond. Ibn Abbas wrote that the prophet said: 'Whoever has many worries and concerns, let him frequently recite *Laa hawla wa la quwwata ill abillah* [there is no power or strength except with Allah]'. 'Whoever persists in praying for forgiveness, Allah will give him a way out of every worry and distress, and will provide for him from sources he could never imagine'. The scribe Usamah ibn Shuraik also wrote about the sayings of the Prophet: 'O Allah's Messenger! Should we seek medical treatment for our illnesses?' He replied: 'Yes, you should seek medical treatment, because God, the Exalted, has let no disease exist without providing for its cure, except for one, namely, death.'

INDIAN HEALING TRADITIONS
Possessing spirits

I conducted original fieldwork in India on medical, religious and spiritual ways of understanding mental health and I interviewed psychiatrists, clairvoyants and religious leaders about the causes of ill health (Tobert 2014). Among South Asian populations, there were many reasons why an individual sufferer may not be 'to blame' for their mental or emotional ill health. For example, if human beings misbehave towards each other, the land or the deities, they can expect to incur the latter's wrath. Deities' anger may strike at either individuals or the group, though it does not necessarily fall on those whose conduct caused it.

In India people agreed that physical and mental illness, childlessness and other misfortunes could be attributed to the spirits of the dead and to *djinn* (entities that had not been incarnate as human). Spirits of the dead (*bhuta*) were spirits of people who had met an 'untimely' death: they were considered not to have passed over to the land of their dead ancestors. These 'ghosts' remained in limbo and populated the places of the living where they inflicted sickness, madness and bad luck. People believed malevolent spirits took possession of the living and controlled their minds and bodies. There was a widespread distinction between 'bad' spirits that possessed their victims and 'good' spirits that possessed diviners or ascetics and gave them clairvoyant skills.

In cases of bad possession, the group may take collective responsibility for the illness of the individual. Exorcism was a public ritual, as it was in Africa, used as a healing therapy during which the sufferer poured out their anger on society or family in a way that was culturally tolerated and would otherwise have been impossible. People who were still alive could cause just as much illness as those who were in spirit: they may be sorcerers or witches or those who unintentionally cast a glance with the 'evil eye' or in jealousy.

SPIRITUAL PSYCHIATRIES

The book *Spiritual Psychiatries* was based on my research in India where I interviewed philosophers, priests and patients. I conducted a qualitative ethnographic research project within the discipline of medical anthropology on mental health-seeking practices.

I discovered in many parts of India that there was no dominant medical paradigm. Patients normally used a plurality of medical therapies concurrently with religious and spiritual practices. When Asian people migrated to the UK, they expected a combination of therapies to be used for their wellbeing.

One psychiatrist I observed had trained in the Cambridge Certificate of Psychiatry at the University of Kolkata. Dr Basu was a devotee of the sage Sri Aurobindo whose ashram was in Pondicherry, South India. In his private practice clinic, he always offered patients the relevant western pharmacological treatments and he might suggest they say prayers at a local temple or shrine. Occasionally he asked clairvoyants or sages for additional spiritual or religious advice about a patient.

In India patients used a multiplicity of treatment strategies, singly, sequentially or contemporaneously. The practitioners consulted included: psychiatrists, psychologists, priests, architectural specialists, clerics, clairvoyants and shamans. They undertook religious rituals – alongside using pharmacological products – to appease the influences of the planets, local deities, the effects of karma or family conflicts. The treatment strategy they selected depended on their theories of illness causation which was influenced by their personal belief system.

In Europe there were also narratives around spirit possession. In 2015, Pope Francis made exorcism an official part of Catholic practice. This gave legal recognition to the performance of liberation or deliverance, used to address some forms of human suffering.

Eastern and Western strategies in India

At the psychiatric clinic there was an acknowledgement that eastern and western beliefs were different and not always compatible. The psychiatrist I spoke to explained that the western model of psychiatry did not fit Indian beliefs about the nature of human existence. General western assumptions were that: we had one life and death was the end; the bodily 'self' was bounded by the skin; mental illness was a condition for life; and, religious rituals were superstitions. In contrast, generalized eastern assumptions were that: we experienced rebirth and repeated incarnations; the bodily 'self' was porous and could be influenced by external forces; mental illness was an episode; and, religion, faith and health were important in daily life.

The topic of dominant models of knowledge was discussed and is summarized below. In the West, for many decades the dominant model of knowledge regarding mental wellbeing was biomedical. Many people assumed western cultural models were ubiquitous (and that others were wrong). However, in India, things were quite different: for example, one man, Professor Katkar, taught philosophy and felt his academic curriculum was culture bound, based on western understandings of the person. He claimed his Indian students were examined according to the knowledge base of another culture. He felt he was teaching philosophy in such a way that it was inappropriate to his students' lives.

On the topic of mental health, he said:

> A system that is termed abnormal in America need not be abnormal here in our culture. These differences exist, within psychiatry, psychology or philosophy. For example hearing music, where no one is playing, may be treated as a symptom of schizophrenia by western psychiatry, but an Indian doctor may think that there is some ghost or spirit in contact with the person. Perhaps we may say that the Indian doctor is unscientific, but his own scientific treatment is Indian, for he may prescribe a lower dose, and it may work. If it works and a person becomes free of their symptoms, this means we need change to a result-oriented outlook. (Tobert 2014, p.241)

Dr Suneet, who taught psychology, continued the conversation:

> the western approach, being the medical model, is based on classification of diseases, with strict categories as found in the DSM. Mostly within the academic world, our students are taught the western model. Somewhere as a footnote, it is mentioned that there are certain Indian approaches. But these approaches are not taken up in detail nor in any systematic manner in our university departments. (p.244)

Both lecturers were frustrated at having to meet western exam board requirements for teaching which did not incorporate their students' life experiences. Academic restrictions placed on scholars in India may be part of colonial blindness or may be part of a deeper western denial about existential and spiritual realities. Furthermore, within the field of mental health, the assertion that biomedical models of interpretation are universal is currently being profoundly challenged.

Professor Katkar, now known as Shrigurudev, explained about psychology and the export of colonial thought and knowledge. He said although India had gained independence in 1947, it did not have independence of thought. The Indian education system accepted teaching colonial psychology and philosophy which were irrelevant to the beliefs of both staff and students.

Alternative remedies

In India, as well as undertaking pilgrimages, people tried other remedies at the same time: for example, homoeopathy has long been used to treat extreme experiences. I found an interesting book in a library in Solapur, Maharashtra. It was by Dr Andre Saine (2004) entitled *Pure Classical Homeopathy: Teaching Psychiatric Patients*. In over 500 or so pages it contained analyses, case studies with follow-up details, diagnoses and homeopathic remedies. Saine was a natural physician who discovered homoeopathy as an effective treatment for mental health in 1976; it offered a more gentle strategy for healing extreme experiences than pharmacology.

Also in India I was introduced to Dr Mahesh who practised psychiatry but also used homoeopathy as a treatment, which he found effective. He eventually stood down from his profession and offered only homoeopathic treatments to his patients. Perhaps practitioners of western psychiatry could consider using homeopathic remedies? At the International Academy of Advanced Homoeopathy in Mumbai where Dr Mahesh teaches, a video is made of each consultation (with consent) to create a huge evidence base of in-depth study and research.

When I conducted research in India for the *Spiritual Psychiatries* book, I discovered there were different ways of interpreting and treating extreme experiences. There were different understandings of consciousness and the self.

THERAPEUTIC COMMUNICATION

The practice of listening topped the list of therapeutic communication styles and it was more important than verbal or non-verbal expression. One university reported that active listening reduced the defensiveness of the client, helping a person assess a situation correctly and avoiding the need to repeat information. It reduced emotions that blocked clear thinking and helped the client feel cared about and understood.

The psychiatrist Arthur Kleinman has suggested heathcare practitioners could use ten questions to engage with a patient and honour them as an expert in their ill health. These were:

- What do you think has caused your problem?

- Why do you think it started when it did?

- What do you think your sickness does to you?

- How does it work?

- How severe is your sickness?

- Will it have a short or long course?

- What kind of treatment do you think you should receive?

- What are the most important results you hope to receive from this treatment?

- What are the chief problems your sickness has caused for you?

- What do you fear most about your sickness?

Kleinman's insight was that clinical reality was considered differently by the doctor and the patient. He said our 'systematic inattention to illness is in part responsible for patient non-compliance, patient and family dissatisfaction with professional healthcare, and inadequate clinical care' (Kleinman *et al.* 1978, p.251). Disease and illness were separate elements of 'sickness', and while disease was a malfunction of the biological system, illness was a sufferer's experience and response to their symptoms.

To what extent do our healthcare organizations have culturally responsive practices and build positive, supportive relationships with staff and patients? Do they help staff make connections with cultural diversity and work well with a patient's family and community? Do our organizations support culturally diverse patients and staff so they collaborate well with other professionals? The issue of spirituality went beyond culture, as we found families of the same culture whose beliefs were radically different; one person was materialist and one spiritualist.

SUMMARY

The question as to what is or isn't a mental health problem is extremely contentious; different cultural groups clearly interpret their conditions and experiences differently. I have explored assumptions around the terms 'knowledge' and 'belief' and have noted that it was usually public consensus that decided.

I have also noted colonial assumptions around what was or wasn't knowledge and the underlying assumption that there was only one way of looking at things. I have presented research from an American university where practitioner beliefs influenced the types of treatments offered to their patients.

This chapter has unpacked and has attempted to discern differences between understanding mental health issues from either an observer's perspective or from a participant's perspective. I have given examples of a range of explanatory models for 'symptoms' from people I have worked with in the UK, India and Africa. There is a deep need to have cultural humility and good listening skills in these times of urban cultural heterogeneity.

13

ANOMALOUS EXPERIENCES

D. Popular Uprisings and Spiritual Awakening

INTRODUCTION

In the previous chapters I have explored experiences that used to come under the catch-all term of 'religious experiences' but which are now referred to as 'spiritual experiences'. I then covered a few examples of NDEs and OBEs. I also presented material on the 'cultural beliefs' of a variety of ethnic groups, data gathered from my own research and from the anthropological literature.

I mentioned all this material because it is my proposition that people experiencing mental health episodes may be having spiritual experiences but cannot switch them off and may become hypersensitive, confused by being caught up in scenarios and visions. In this chapter I take a deeper look at spontaneous experiences: those that occur by chance but which cannot be stopped at will.

There are many ways of interpreting these experiences. I mentioned at the start of this book that many years ago I received an insight indicating that spiritual experiences and mental health were on a continuum. Today, this view is expressed by many people on social media sites and has even made an appearance in the academic literature (Clarke 2010, Gale *et al.* 2014). It also features in the popular press, online blogs and in interviews with spiritual seekers. My own article on anomalous experiences was recently published in a journal in India, on New Approaches to Medicine and Health (Tobert 2016).

Cultural psychiatrists have also noted that there are many ways of interpreting the evidence of symptoms (Littlewood and Dein 2001). This is important from several people's perspectives which need to be taken into account: the cultural views of new migrants and the cultural views of people possessing spiritual beliefs about health.

In today's world, there is no longer binary knowledge; there is no longer a true or false way of understanding health. There is a plurality of explanations for ill health and not simply one single truth.

It is important to know about people's existential beliefs about their experiences because these influence explanatory models for certain symptoms of distress and affect access to healthcare and compliance with treatment.

The contents of this chapter include social media and the popular uprising of sufferers. I also discuss extreme experiences and spiritual awakening. I will cover the practice of Open Dialogue treatment which is gaining global momentum and creating changes in clinical practice.

POPULAR UPRISING OF SUFFERERS
Extreme experiences

Extreme experiences may also be called spiritual crises or spiritual emergencies. People may feel as though they are receiving too much visual or auditory information which becomes unmanageable or distressing. They may feel enhanced awareness or that they have clairvoyant skills, as if their mind is being bombarded with inner experiences. They may feel out of touch with ordinary reality.

With good support, sufferers often find experiences profoundly transformative. However, relatives may have different beliefs about extreme experiences. They may think a person has had a breakdown or mental health problems or they may take the event as indicative of schizophrenia.

However, people from non-industrial societies may have a different reaction. They may assume the experiences are altered states of consciousness which offer insights into reincarnation, spirit possession or shamanic journeying. The same experiences may be interpreted in different ways by different professions and this is a problem.

If the people around the experient are calm and have a belief system which fits, they can offer appropriate measures. The problem lies, however, when some psychiatrists identify such human experiences as indicative of pathology, schizophrenia or psychosis. When force is used on a sufferer, they may respond with violence.

Psychologists (Bentall *et al.* 2014) have started to rise up against the medical model of psychosis and schizophrenia, with the support of the International Association of Near-Death Studies and the International Society for Psychological and Social Approaches to Psychosis. Online blogs and interviews abound and the mainstream media followed later.

Mental health and spiritual awakening

Today there is an angry uprising against western psychiatry across the world. People who were diagnosed with psychosis and schizophrenia are questioning their diagnosis and treatment. With the help of the internet, Facebook, Twitter and blogging, the survivor movement has swelled. People can compare diagnoses and their treatments. They can rise up quickly against any action taken that they do not feel is appropriate.

There appeared to be different stages leading towards this change. First, there was grief at the lost years due to perceived overmedication, followed by profound anger, then a determined movement to raise awareness and support other 'service users'. There is now a dynamic move towards changing mainstream diagnosis and treatment and integrating new paradigm practices.

Psychiatrists themselves have questioned diagnosis, for example Russell Razzaque (2014) suggested that experiences may be part of a spiritual awakening, part of a journey of transformation. Likewise his colleague, Katie Mottram (2014), had her own spiritual awakening. She wants to address the pathologizing of mental distress and has vowed to bring about changes in mental healthcare.

Although much material about change was publically available on social media, the mental health education of medical students continued along old-fashioned historical tracks. The older views of 'diseases of the brain' and 'chemical imbalances' were deeply embedded in education, both in medical and healthcare providers and in the lay public.

When I taught medical anthropology courses in medical schools, setting out the psycho/social/environmental triggers for mental distress, students tried to correct me, as they had just be taught a rather racist version of ethnic predispositions. Students believed in the old teachings of the predispositions of this or that ethnic group towards psychosis. Their educators offered a racist perspective, in denial about the historical, social or environmental triggers of distress. I felt they needed to consider change and modernization but I was unsure how to mobilize radical change in the education system.

I realized really close friends of mine, who were healthcare providers, rigorously trained in this older way thinking, held onto their beliefs about psychosis, pharmacology and ECT treatments. I tried to open the door to dialogue.

CHANGES IN PRACTICE
Spiritual perspectives in the West

In 2016, many people who had been within the psychiatric system claimed their experience was a spiritual awakening. This resulted from a fundamental belief that certain types of mental distress were spiritual emergencies. In the last few years, a flurry of publications has suggested this. Katie Mottram had an extreme experience which shook the very foundations of her understanding of the world. She claimed this was part of her spiritual awakening. She had worked within mental health for 15 years and she recounted her personal story of growing up with her mother who had been pathologized by the psychiatric system. Catherine Lucas (2011) presented a book with narratives about spiritual emergencies and then offered a set of guidelines to survive them.

Both acknowledged the need to engage with both the psychiatric and the spiritual worlds. Katie's mission was to normalize extreme experiences within mainstream society so they became more widely acknowledged within the psychiatric system. She was also involved in a national mental health service pilot project (Peer-Supported Open Dialogue) and offered support to establish an International Spiritual Emergency Network (ISEN). Her long-term aim was to support education initiatives which would help alleviate mental distress. She was a member of the UK Spiritual Crisis Network (SCN).

Isabel Clarke was a clinical psychologist, working in acute mental health in the NHS, who established the SCN. She noted that the preoccupation of people experiencing psychotic breakdowns with religious ideas was not mysterious. She recognized that a person having extreme experiences needed support and practical assistance and she offered a fundamental rethink of the concept of psychosis and proposed new insights into spirituality. She set up an online moderated email service for people who had had experiences – the psychosis spirituality support group – which became very popular. She was also instrumental in supporting the Revisioning Mental Health Group, supported by Catherine Lucas.

In the UK, one psychiatrist who worked in the NHS in East London had a special interest in mindfulness which he had practised for years. He was particularly interested in understanding consciousness and its connection between spirituality and mental health. In his book, he explored new insights into the mind and mental distress. His conclusion was that mental illness, to which he acknowledged everyone was susceptible, could be a form of spiritual awakening (Razzaque 2014). Today he is researching a new form of mental health provision – Open Dialogue.

USA initiatives

In 2015 a new online platform was set up on Facebook by Dabney Alix who described herself as a spiritual business coach, visionary and naturopath. Called Shades of Awakening, this online platform was also a closed group, supporting people who'd had extreme experiences. Her aim was to offer genuine validation for those who had had spiritual awakenings, while suggesting visitors sought professional medical advice.

Shades quickly attracted over 2500 people and became a community interested in spiritual emergencies, awakenings and contemporary alternatives to mental health diagnoses and treatment. Their mission statement is: 'We believe that extreme states of consciousness, often considered by psychiatry to be pathological, can be transformative and part of [a] personal and planetary awakening.'

The website quickly drew a huge international following and supported its participants in acknowledging and offering re-interpretations of experience. It was enormously supportive and valuable for the social acknowledgement of followers. People shared their own 'anomalous' experiences and this offered support to those who, up until then, had only received a pathological response to their condition.

Also in the USA, there was the transpersonal psychologist Emma Bragdon, founder of Integrative Mental Health for You (IMHU) which provided online courses for health professionals with experts in various fields. Emma had visited Brazil and observed the work of spiritist psychiatrists first hand. Her organization focused on psychological and social support for people who experienced problems, as well as nutrition and lifestyle advice. It offered teaching via online webinars, courses and interviews.

TED talks were established in California in the 1980s and they continued, even though one by the biologist Rupert Sheldrake (2013) on the belief system of science was banned. The spiritual author Eckhart Tolle has grown in prominence and his online seminars on the challenges of life and suffering have had a huge following. The physician Larry Dossey has suggested there was a limit to scientific knowledge and our beliefs influenced how we interpreted extreme experiences (2015). He explored the ways in which materialist explanations for consciousness failed and suggested there was evidence that consciousness transcended physicalism (that everything which existed did not go beyond its physical properties).

Beliefs about the validity of anomalous experiences do seem to come from a different existential paradigm and they seem to influence how we interpret extreme experiences. The transpersonal psychologist David Lukoff (2007) gave an explanation to address the relationship between mystical experiences and psychosis. He was instrumental in working with the producers of the DSM-IV to ensure the category of spirituality was included. The Spiritual Competency Resource Centre he established offers access to web-based resources to encourage the cultural sensitivity of mental health professionals. The topic is accepted as a key part of cultural competence for mental health professionals.

Open Dialogue

In the UK, consultant psychiatrist Russell Razzaque spearheaded a movement for change in the NHS. Trained in psychology and mindfulness, and interested in the study of consciousness, he was involved in researching its use in adult mental health. He and Nick Putnam were practising supporters of Open Dialogue, an approach used in Finland with people experiencing a mental health crisis and their families.

Steps are being taken to engage with mainstream medical and healthcare professionals in North East London to promote these practices and train staff in new ways of addressing extreme experiences. A number of NHS Trusts are discussing Open Dialogue, and the North East London Foundation Trust (NELFT) organized a well attended national conference on developing Peer-Supported Open Dialogue (POD).

A new (ancient) way of working with people with first episode psychosis problems was promoted. I put ancient in brackets, as the way problems used to be solved in Africa, indigenous America and Australia was by a gerontocracy, a meeting of elders who practised open dialogue. In the UK and the USA, the Soteria network promoted therapeutic environments with a minimum of drugs for people who experienced extreme states of consciousness. In Finland, where Open Dialogue became the main psychiatric treatment practice, the originators demonstrated through research that this strategy reduced hospitalization, the use of medication and relapse (Seikkula *et al.* 2006).

The seed of the idea for Open Dialogue started in the UK around 2003 and was adapted from family therapy – the winds of change have been blowing ever since. Psychiatrists began exploring new paradigms for addressing mental distress. The first pilot using Open Dialogue was run in 2015, with participants from four NHS trusts being taught new ways of addressing mental distress. They said the training was transformational.

I co-facilitated a day's training in Birmingham for four NHS trusts which supported an Open Dialogue UK approach. The topic was on cultural diversity and spiritual awakening. We continued to offer workshops to NHS trusts on mental wellbeing and spiritual experiences.

We had a number of aims: to acknowledge the current dilemma around the interpretation of symptoms; to invite staff to work with a client's spiritual and religious beliefs; to raise awareness of the cultural expressions of mental distress; and, to deepen the awareness of cultural and religious explanatory models for diagnosis and treatment.

After a conference in London, it felt like the tide was turning and attitudes were changing. There were plans for the training to continue with a new cohort of participants from more NHS trusts. Meetings were held with the Department of Health and officials towards a nationwide transformation of service provision.

There was also interest in Japan in Open Dialogue. In 2015, around 50 people participated in a meeting, including staff from 15 different universities, psychiatrists, psychologists, researchers, PhD students and medical journalists.

A WAY FORWARD
Where do we go from here?

In my opinion, there is no single truth. The duality between knowledge and belief no longer exists. Now there appears to be a plurality of beliefs and practices. In addition, it appears that some individuals are so sensitive that they can access visionary experiences without taking any substances, just by intending to focus. My interest lies in those people who have spontaneous experiences and appear to be diagnosed as 'schizophrenic' by those observers who do not have spiritual frameworks of understanding.

I don't believe in the predispositions of this or that ethnic group to psychosis. That seems to be a very narrow assumption. I believe it is a normal human function to have these experiences. That is everyone, indeed anyone, can open the doors of perception or have them opened. Triggers may include the use of substances like ayahuasca or childhood traumas, past life traumas, present life traumas, forced migration or shamanic drumming. For some people, they are quite simply born with the doors of perception open.

They are born psychic, clairvoyant or clairsentient. If people around them are aware of this, they are supported. If not, then due to a combination of factors, they may find themselves given a label or a diagnosis. These are my beliefs. I would like to see a research project comparing the phenomenology of each type of experience with the aim of challenging old-fashioned diagnoses.

My proposition is that each of these spiritual experiences is an example of expanded consciousness which is spontaneous, sought or cannot be turned off. I assume that all human beings have a normal in-built capacity to have 'anomalous' experiences, if not during their life, then at the end of their life.

How can we address the dilemma between old educational beliefs and current healthcare practice in hospitals and medical centres? How can we change the consensus on human experiences to be more inclusive? And how can we set hospital protocols according to a wider perspective of consciousness? I will explore these matters in the final two chapters.

SUMMARY

In this chapter I have explored social media and the popular uprising of sufferers. I have also discussed extreme experiences and spiritual awakening and have noted the uprising of psychotherapists against the medical model of distress. I have covered the innovative practice of Open Dialogue which is gaining global momentum. I have also looked at shifting belief systems around altered states of consciousness, reality and human experience.

In the following chapter I will propose that there is a spiritual dimension which some people access deliberately and some by chance. Some people are disturbed by it and have no framework for understanding their experiences. I will present those people who deliberately choose to access altered states of consciousness.

14

ANOMALOUS EXPERIENCES

E. Deliberate Shifts in Consciousness

In this chapter I will look at those people who have made deliberate attempts to shift consciousness in order to access visionary or auditory states. I also mention specialists who invoke experiences by intention or by engaging with specific practices.

HOW DO WE DEFINE OUR EXPERIENCES?
What is the issue?

Human beings have had religious experiences since time immemorial, from Moses and the burning bush to Florence Nightingale hearing the word of God. In recent times, the term 'religious experiences' has been replaced by 'spiritual experiences'. Some people, like Taylor (2016), suggest that psychosis is similar but different to spiritual awakening, while others suggest it is on a continuum.

Whatever the terms mean, the experiences appear to be on a continuum with spiritual emergencies and mental health's perception of visionary and auditory experiences. These experiences can be transformative but spiritual experiences tend to start and stop. Pathology is invoked when people cannot stop the phenomena. The question is whether it is a normal human faculty to have such experiences.

What is normal?

The proposition: the explanatory model we chose for those experiences, the way we interpreted the phenomena, depended on our belief system about the nature of reality, influenced by the common consensus view of our cultural background and our peers.

What are normal human experiences? Unusual and anomalous experiences can be superficially divided in three groups: those experiences which are benevolent and occur spontaneously; those which are deliberately sought by specialists; and, those which are negative and may result in a mental health diagnosis. Other professions may have other terms for identifying these experiences but this is what I have chosen.

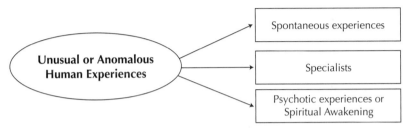

Figure 14.1. Anomalous Human Experiences

The Canadian physician Gabor Mate (2014) gave an interview for the *Crazywise* film on the nature of 'normal'. He noted that the best place to have psychosis was in villages in India or Africa where people supported a sufferer. In the West, he said the event was a 'culturally manufactured, culturally constructed paradigm' where sufferers were separated from spirituality and society (2014).

Spontaneous experiences may include religious or mystical experiences, visions, transcendence, presences, sudden clairvoyance, OBEs, ELEs and NDEs. These experiences are not sought but may occur to a human being in any setting.

These kinds of experience may not be unusual or anomalous to those specialists who deliberately seek them out, either professionals like traditional doctors, healers, shamans, psychics, mediums, seers and clairvoyants, or those who seek them on purpose by consuming substances, engaging in trance dance or drumming.

Psychotic experiences appear to be similar but with either a negative content or a deeply negative effect on the experient that is assumed to be 'abnormal' by those around them. These include people experiencing psychosis, voices, visions and those who have no on/off switch to stop the experience.

Some people appear spontaneously to switch dimensions into spiritual realms and do not have an explanatory framework for their experience. They may become confused and distressed. They may carry out negative actions that they claim are influenced by 'other-than-human-beings'. In association with other factors, this may result in a psychiatric diagnosis

Having an out-of-body or near-death experience is transformative and may deeply affect people, both the experients and those around them (e.g. relatives, healthcare professionals and religious practitioners). However, the response to those experiences may depend on whether or not the observer is familiar with them, rather than the experience in its own right. That is, responses may be impromptu.

What is unusual or anomalous?

There seems to be an ambiguity as to the boundaries between spiritual experience and mental health. In theory it is clear, in practice it is not. The question as to what is considered normal or abnormal is open to discussion. The psychologist, Rosenhan, from Stanford University wrote: 'What is or is not normal may have much to do with the labels that are applied to people in particular settings.' Rosenhan carried out an experiment (which ethics would not allow today) to explore the validity of psychiatric diagnoses – he concluded: 'It is clear that we cannot distinguish the sane from the insane in psychiatric hospitals' (1973, p.398).

On the topic of anomalous human experiences, Karl Osis (1961, p.164), director of the American Society of Psychic Research, wrote:

> In the West if a discarnate being should appear to the recently bereaved as a hallucination or apparition this may be considered delusional or a case of 'complicated grief', whereas in other societies it might be a welcome vision.

Today, having exceptional, anomalous or extreme experiences appears to be normal, as part of every human being's faculties, depending on their history and circumstances. Recent online published articles, such as in the *Journal of Exceptional Experiences and Psychology*, are now available. Parapsychologists like David Luke (2012) have compared the phenomenology of extreme experiences with those of the paranormal. His colleague, Jack Hunter, has also written extensively on other dimensions and has suggested that nature itself is multidimensional.

Similarly, Christian de Quincey (2015) has spoken on panpsychism and consciousness and has explored the nature of being and the nature of reality. He explained that matter and mind went together, so consciousness was embodied. Panpsychism was the belief that all material things held an aspect of consciousness.

VISIONARY EXPERIENCES

The American writer, Joseph Rael, had a series of visionary experiences when he was a child. In church with his grandfather, he watched 'angelic beings created by the energy of prayer'. When he walked about the pueblo, he saw it as it was thousands of years ago. He saw rivers and mountains forming, and watched as katchina figures descended and transformed into stone (Rael 2012). In his society, among the indigenous American people of Picuris Pueblo, visions were not only normal, but sought after.

Interdimensional specialists

In this section I consider spontaneous experiences which start, occur and stop. I am interested in this because if these phenomena are veridical, we need to compare them with the visionary experiences of those who may suffer a psychosis event. Below I briefly address clairvoyance, mediumship and shamanic journeying, each of which is deliberately invoked. Figure 14.2 illustrates the polarities of human consciousness.

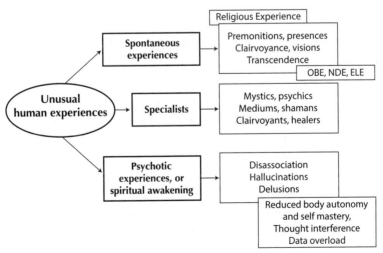

Figure 14.2. Unusual Human Experiences: Polarities of Consciousness

Spiritualists and clairvoyants

There are a series of experiential practices that can bridge the realms of consciousness between health, life and death. Most societies have specialists who claim to be interdimensionally clairvoyant: that is they see, talk to or negotiate with the spirits of the dead. In the West they are called psychics or mediums, elsewhere they may be known as shamans, although their functions regarding consciousness and wellbeing are different. Mediums are people who receive communications from beings in the non-physical realm.

Those who attend spiritualist churches believe a medium is a messenger bringing information to a person in the physical world. Spiritualists believe that the soul can leave the body at will, while the spirit resides in the body and leaves on death. This is similar to the Lelet of Melanesia mentioned earlier, who consider human consciousness and the body as inseparable: once a person dies the body decomposes, and the life force permanently separates from the body via the fontanel. The life force is not considered to be immaterial because it can be seen after death, but during life it is invisible.

A clairvoyant may see spirits: objectively or with his or her eyes open, or subjectively through their soul (perhaps with their eyes closed). Messages interpreted as coming from the dead have been in vogue for spiritualists since the mid-nineteenth century. The Professor of Theology and Religious Studies, Paul Badham, has claimed that cases of contact with the deceased have been recorded since the fourth century CE.

Mediumship and contact with the dead

In the past, contact with a deceased person either visually or through words was frequently considered to be either a hallucination or evidence that the person in question was delusional.

Professor Paul Badham taught at the department of religious studies at University of Wales in Lampeter. He has claimed there was a strong case for the existence of extrasensory perception; if thoughts could pass from one brain to another in the living, it may be possible for there to be communication between the living and the dead.

If there was such a thing as life after death, thoughts could be passed telepathically into an embodied human being. In this way, the stream of consciousness could be perceived to continue after death. Badham (1997) suggested there were numerous cases and it would be better to consider them as 'veridical'. He said such cases had been recorded since the fourth century CE. He suggested there may be dual states of existence: materialist and psychic.

However, his colleague, the Christian pastor Paul Edwards (1997) claimed that the supposition there is a 'non-physical storage depot of extra-cerebral memories…must surely be dismissed as nothing but a vague picture which is of no scientific value whatsoever.' There are extremely diverse views about issues of survival, even by clergy.

Shamanic journey

Shamans are people who can master discarnate spirits and introduce them at will into their own body. A shaman is a man or woman who intentionally communicates with the non-physical realms. They undertake a journey to other worlds for various reasons: on behalf of others, for the community, to gain information about environmental resources or to effect healing. They work with 'other-than-human-beings' (Harvey 2002, p.10).

Shamanic journeys require an individual to deliberately undertake a visualization or lucid dream with the intention of finding out or healing something for themselves or the benefit of others. The experiencer intentionally enters into an altered state of consciousness using drumming, drugs or certain body postures. They claim to alter their bodily frequency, transcend space and time and engage in a kind of remote viewing in non-physical realms, seeing ancestral spirits and doing psychopomp work (i.e. helping those who have died a violent death resolve the issues and transform into an ancestral spiritual dimension).

These specialists deliberately seek out-of-body experiences and also experience a non-corporeal, non-local centre of perception. In the West, the interest in neo-shamanism has greatly increased over the last couple of decades. This is an experiential practice which was originally influenced by indigenous American and African traditions.

Although nowadays it is more common in the West for psychics and mediums to remain silent about what they do or do not see in spirit realms, those who undertake experiential shamanic journeys have a wide following, with journals devoted to the practice and many books published on personal empowerment and environmental healing (Rutherford 2008, Villoldo 2015b).

When I conducted the research project at Brunel University mentioned in Chapter 10, I explored the testimonies of respondents who had had experiences. Out of sixty responses, 45 people said they had deliberately undertaken practices which they believed might result in an altered state experience. The most popular practice was meditation (43% of respondents), followed by shamanic practices and visualization techniques (15% of the total).

Many found their practices were transformational and promoted healing; they felt empowered and their lives were enriched (Tobert 2000). People used different strategies to deliberately shift into altered states of consciousness and these included consuming substances (legal and illegal), trance dancing and repetitive beat shamanic drumming.

If these altered states of consciousness can be invoked at will, are they similar to psychotic experiences, and if they are, might it be possible to invite an experient to witness their uncontrolled event and negotiate with them to manage it?

Remote viewing and military psychics

In the USA, organizations have been established since the 1970s, such as the Monroe Institute, where people could learn how to deliberately have an out-of-body or remote viewing experience. The Russians have been interested in this phenomenon since the 1920s, possibly for military purposes (Morehouse 2000).

The information below on remote viewing may or may not be accurate as it was taken from social media sources. However, I am interested in it because if remote viewing is veridical, it may be that people experiencing psychosis, anomalous vents or spiritual awakening may be sensitively tuning in like a radio frequency to information from other places. Having no framework for understanding, they may become confused by it.

Both the US military and the Russian military have supposedly used remote viewing as a safe way of collecting data, although apparently it was not always sanctioned by those in high command. In the US, there was a remote viewing laboratory at the Stanford Research Institute which was used by the military. The US government had used scientific remote viewing to collect information about their country's perceived enemies since the 1970s. In 1995 the CIA declassified a top-secret programme which had trained people in remote viewing and explored the human capacity to transcend time and space (Zutshi 2012). They claimed it was not effective.

In 1982 a set of protocols was developed by Ingo Swann whereby remote viewing was based on geographical coordinates to explore a given target. People were trained in out-of-body-states at the Monroe Institute in Virginia. Remote viewing of earth-based sites could be independently confirmed: the data was either accurate or not. Today there are several organizations that offer training like the Farsight Institute and the Remote Viewing Instructional Services (RVIS).[1]

If remote viewing can be invoked at will, according to a set of controlled coordinates, does the practice have any relationship with psychotic experiences? If it does, might it be possible to invite an experient to witness their uncontrolled event and with compassion negotiate with them to manage it?

Paranormal experiences

There is renewed interest in the paranormal: events and phenomena that cannot yet be explained by the laws of nature and which appear to lie beyond scientific knowledge. However, the parapsychologist Carlos Alvarado (2014, 2015) has suggested 'paranormal' experiences were a normal part of human psychology and noted there was much parapsychology research conducted on healing.

At Northampton University, research was conducted into non-contact healing (Roe *et al.* 2015). Their Centre for the Study of Anomalous Psychological Processes explored the nature of anomalous experiences and also undertook research into life after death. During an interview with the transpersonal psychologist Charles Tart (2015), he spoke about human existence, transpersonal experience and parapsychological research.

In Europe, the International Society for Psychological and Social Approaches to Psychosis (ISPS) started in Switzerland in the 1950s. It promoted psychotherapy and psychological treatments for people who had psychosis or who had been diagnosed with 'schizophrenia'; their intention was to collaborate with mainstream health practitioners and service users.

---

1   http://farsight.org/learning.html and www.rviewer.com

The psychologist, David Luke, has explored the intersection between altered states of consciousness and anomalous psychological phenomena (2013). Likewise Jack Hunter had similar research interests: contemporary trance and physical mediumship, focusing on personhood, altered states of consciousness and anomalous experience. He established the journal *Paranthropology* to explore anthropological approaches to the paranormal to promote the dialogue on paranormal beliefs, experiences and phenomena. His book, edited with David Luke, addresses the phenomenology of spirits in global settings (2014).

Human understanding of existential reality varies widely, as examples in earlier chapters of this book have suggested. Furthermore, the discipline of medical anthropology illustrates that what is normal in one society may be considered abnormal in another.

There have been anthropologists who have looked at shamanism and psychedelia experiences; for example, Fiona Bowie (2002, 2013) did research on anthropologists who had experiences which they couldn't compute, as did Goulet and Miller (2007), and David Luke and Jack Hunter reported on psychedelics and spiritism. Other parapsychologists have reviewed the scientific evidence for anomalous experiences (Cardeña *et al.* 2004).

Today, there are extensive reading lists on research undertaken on psychic phenomena. The parapsychologist, Dean Radin, has selected a set of peer-reviewed publications on PSI research. A selection of such articles is available online and is downloadable. The majority were published in the twenty-first century. This is a marvellous resource.

Thin places

What is the relevance of the above material to mental health? Is it possible that people who experience psychosis might be sensitive to the paranormal? Is it possible that they might experience a 'thin' place between the worlds where their person can be overshadowed by paranormal activity?

The Celtic peoples in ancient Britain believed a 'thin' place was where humans could experience dimensions of transcendence or divinity between heaven and earth. For some people, their experiences may feel as if they are between heaven and hell. Madeleine Gray, professor of Ecclesiastic History, suggested at a meeting of the Scientific and Medical Network that a 'thin place' was between locations in this world where a person could transcend space and time (2011).

I wanted to explore whether it was possible for professionals from different academic disciplines to sit round a table and discuss with each other the phenomenology of experiences (Tobert 2015b). I gave a talk in San Francisco on anomalous experiences and cultural interpretations where I presented spiritual explanatory models for experiences and discussed eastern and western frameworks of knowledge. I wanted to explore how we might encourage positive change in attitudes towards mental healthcare practice.

WHAT IS THE NATURE OF BEING HUMAN?

These discussions about specialists and other people who spontaneously have visionary or spiritual experiences seem to beg the question: why are some individuals pathologized? It seemed that so many people could deliberately or spontaneously go into an altered state of consciousness that it appeared like a normal practice. Are not the phenomena very similar, but some are contained, whilst others are not contained very well? Sometimes intervention appeared to depend on the framework of understanding of both the experient and the observer.

Existential paradigms

It seemed our beliefs about the nature of reality affected our understanding and interpretation of this group of 'religious experiences'. Our beliefs about the nature of human existence and consciousness beyond death appeared to influence our judgement and the boundaries of accepted knowledge or research topics.

It is possible that, for some people, their frameworks of knowledge influenced the diagnosis and treatment of certain types of mental distress. I mentioned the Testimony Project in Chapter 7, which consisted of in-depth interviews with long-term inmates of twentieth-century psychiatric institutions. The triggers of distress seemed to belong to mundane happenings in the patients' lives and yet they found themselves incarcerated in institutions for things common consensus would not accept today. Society has already started another cultural U-turn in the way these experiences are treated.

Over time, as humans we have changed our beliefs and we have modified or adapted our responses to anomalous or religious experiences (or out-of-body experiences or end-of-life experiences or near-death experiences).

One explanatory model is that religious experience tapped into a dimension, beyond the five senses, which some people accessed deliberately, some by chance, and yet others accessed it but were traumatized and confused it with 'common consensus reality'. They could not witness what was happening.

POLARITIES OF CONSCIOUSNESS

Co-existing belief systems concern:

- the nature of human experience
- the nature of reality

Cultural and popular explanatory models:

- Transcendence – experience of the numinous or mystical, both beyond and incorporating the self

- Dissociation – the body stays in same place, but the centre of perception appears to wander independently

- Remote viewing – body stays within same time, but consciousness, or the centre of perception moves to 'other places', or travels between various geographical locations and time frames

- Presence – angels, guides, spirits of the dead are seen, body and consciousness exist at the same time and place, but tune into spiritual dimensions

- Past life memory – the body stays in same place, but centre of perception perceives 'other time frames'

- Spirit possession – the body of a human being is 'porous', and is overshadowed by human and non-human entities

- Voices are heard – the body is porous and live and dead beings can verbally assault, or assist, the individual

- Psychosis – spiritual dimensions are accessed by accident; they are confused with 'common-consensus reality', and the individual can not find the on/off switch

UNDERLYING ASSUMPTIONS

- a spiritual dimension exists some access it deliberately; some by chance; others are disturbed by it, and have no framework for understanding their experience.

Figure 14.3. The Polarities of Consciousness

Shifting belief systems

Perhaps it is time to re-evaluate the meaning behind some terms which are commonly used? Figure 14.3 illustrates the polarities of consciousness. The way we use words and interpret data seems to change over time. According to dictionary definitions, 'to hallucinate' is to see something which is not there or it may be to see something which other people say is not there. Common consensus has decided it is a hallucination.

Likewise a 'delusion' is a false belief, an error or a hallucination but it could also be a belief which other people disagree with. A vision is something seen by a mystic, or a sighting which other people accept has occurred. Veridical means telling the truth, coinciding with fact that is, it is agreed that something corresponded to what happened.

While an apparition is something startling which some people may believe has appeared and some may not, it may be considered to be veridical. Each of these interpretations of the above words depends on the common consensus of one's peers or colleagues. It does not seem as though there is a fixed interpretation unless other indicators (or symptoms) are present.

SUMMARY

I have explored the definitions of normal experiences and suggested that having certain experiences was a normal part of the human condition. I noted that the problem arose when some people were pathologized for having experiences when they could not turn off at will, while other experiences were regarded as the normal skills of certain specialists who could travel between dimensions.

I presented specialists (like clairvoyant, psychics and mediums) who deliberately accessed inter-dimensional realms, those who experienced spontaneous non-corporeal consciousness, and those who deliberately chose to put themselves into an altered state as a shaman or as a remote viewer.

I would like to suggest that people from indigenous, non-industrialized societies may have had an awareness of subtle states of consciousness which, in the early days of data collection, may have been regarded as 'superstitious' but which in today's modern world may be regarded as having deep insights into altered states of consciousness.

In the following chapter I will explore the fixed nature of some academic thinking around human experiences and phenomenology and its disinclination to consider mental health or spiritual awakening.

15

WHY ADDRESS CULTURAL UNDERSTANDINGS AND ACADEMIC FIXITY?

OVERVIEW

In this section I will explore why we need to consider having a more profound grasp of cultural understanding and I will look at the interpretations of equalities which appear to have become unconsciously narrow. I explore academic consensus about the terms and phenomenology around spiritual experiences. Finally, I present one theory of change and look at what steps we might take towards a way forwards.

There appears to be a fundamental paradigm divide between those people who maintain a materialist view of life and those who hold a spiritist perspective of existence. The chasm between these two opinions or beliefs about life influences how people interpret anomalous experiences, or whether indeed they refer to experiences as 'anomalous' at all. There are also competing narratives between academic education and information from social media.

If we subtly discount other people's ideas as false, irrational or culture-bound beliefs, how might this influence our interactions with patients? The explanations we select to understand 'anomalous' concepts depend on our own belief system about the nature of human existence and reality. This is influenced by the agreed consensus view of our cultural background. However, as I pointed out in Chapter 7, common consensus is not necessarily right, nor does it withstand the test of time. It may be taken as correct at one point in time, but historical hindsight may suggest actions taken were in poor judgement and needed to be reassessed and apologised for.

WHY ADDRESS CULTURAL UNDERSTANDINGS?

I have discussed the way our beliefs influence our interpretation of mental health. I have covered not only different ways of interpreting mental wellbeing, but also different beliefs about spiritual awakening, survival beyond death and individuals who deliberately seek visionary and auditory experiences.

Our patients and clients may have beliefs that we do not hold. Beliefs in reincarnation and karma may have an influence on a person's health-seeking strategies and whether or not they will accept medication or other treatments. They may consider their illness as fate which they would not want to take through with them into the next life and so they endure it in this one.

In the World Health Organization publication by the health and human rights advisor Nygren-Krug (2001), the importance of cultural competency and shared understandings was emphasized. She explained that our modern health service needs to account for different beliefs in order to be sufficiently culturally sensitive so as not to deny access to or exclude ethnic minorities.

There are two issues regarding mental health: one is cultural humility towards the beliefs of every ethnic group and the other is to suspend judgement about spiritual interpretations.

Culture and communication

The psychiatrist and anthropologist, Arthur Kleinman, has suggested there may be a chasm between doctors' and patients' understandings of the symptoms of illness and sickness. He put forward a series of questions which would enable the client to present their view:

> The wording of questions will vary with characteristics of the patient, the problem, and the setting, but we suggest the following set of questions to elicit the patient explanatory model. Patients often hesitate to disclose their models to doctors. Clinicians need to be persistent in order to show patients that their ideas are of genuine interest and importance for clinical management. (Kleinman, Eisenberg, and Good 1978, p.256)

One way to encourage cultural humility and determine a patient's beliefs would be to use Kleinman's eight questions or other tools of enquiry. These would illicit what the patient believed had caused their illness, their hopes about treatment and their current fears about progression. In this way one can combine clinical and social expertise about the nature of the patient's experience of sickness and medical aspects of disease.

If we were asked to develop a set of protocols surrounding the influence of beliefs on survival beyond death in a clinic with a multicultural population, what issues would we mention? What recommendations would we make to hospital policy makers and managers? How would we be explicit about the underlying assumptions that are present in each culture? How might we acknowledge the boundaries of our own belief systems?

In the UK, the Equality Act has taken on a narrow focus and barely mentions culture and health. There are a multiplicity of ways of understanding life, health and death and a plurality of cultural knowledge frameworks for understanding human existence, life and death. It is essential to understand the many ways of addressing human experience. Culture is not invisible.

NARROW INTERPRETATIONS OF EQUALITIES

The practice of religion and religious rituals is important for societal wellbeing. However, societal problems may occur if service provider organizations focus only on religion (the prayers, rituals, food, feasts, fasts and festivals) and do not engage with 'belief' when trying to adhere to the UK Equality Act. Attending to religion or religious practice alone is an extremely narrow interpretation of equalities and is particularly a problem in healthcare.

Moving equalities

In the UK, we have taken action, or at least one government department conducted research and produced a Delivering Race Equalities (DoH 2005) five-year plan for addressing race equalities and mental health. But what did we do once we had recorded what was happening? RawOrg has suggested that the goals of DRE were fine but they were not delivered (2011).

For example, one DRE goal was to reduce the high detention rates of African groups and minority ethnic groups, as the detention rate under section 37/41 was higher for them than average. However, the five years between the two Count Me In censuses (2005, 2010) showed that 'The overall proportion of patients from minority ethnic groups increased from 20% to 23%' (CQC 2011, p.32). Admission rates and detention were higher than average among minority ethnic groups and admission was six times higher than average (ibid., p.42).

Not once in 2016 did I hear culture or ethnicity mentioned. However, the group of specialists collaborating over the Putting the Soul Back into Psychiatry Report had suggested that 'the most effective way to empower service users is to provide greater choice of therapeutic and other interventions – so psychiatry becomes a gateway to services and one option among others' (Mind 2007). Another goal, though it did not happen immediately. However, with Open Dialogue being accepted as a strategy for addressing mental health within the NHS, it is becoming more possible today.

Different interpretations

People in one culture interpret episodes differently from others. There has been research on this: for example, Tanya Luhrmann wrote that Americans who heard voices assumed they were 'psychotic' but the author made an interesting point that other cultures assumed their voices were spiritual or social manifestations which had more benign outcomes. She appeared to suggest the term 'schizophrenia' was culturally determined (Parker 2014).

Luhrmann, a professor of anthropology at Stanford University, studied how culture affected the experiences of people who had auditory hallucinations, specifically in India, Ghana and the United States. She found that the voice-hearing experiences of people with serious psychotic disorders were shaped by local culture; in the USA, the voices were harsh and threatening, whereas in Africa and India, they were more benign and playful.

One new approach has claimed it was possible to improve individuals' relationships with their voices by teaching them to name them and build relationships with them, and that doing so diminished their caustic qualities: 'Instead, the difference seems to be that the Chennai (India) and Accra (Ghana) participants were more comfortable interpreting their voices as relationships and not as the sign of a violated mind.'

The author noted that:

[m]any in the Chennai and Accra samples seemed to experience their voices as people: the voice was that of a human the participant knew, such as a brother or a neighbor, or a human-like spirit whom the participant also knew. These respondents seemed to have real human relationships with the voices – sometimes even when they did not like them. (Luhrmann *et al.* 2015)

One Dutch psychiatrist, Dr Marius Romme, supported the Hearing Voices Movement during the 1980s. He believed that 'anti-psychotic medication prevented the emotional processing and therefore healing, of the meaning of the voices' (2011). He maintained schizophrenia was not a disease of the brain, rather it was just a part of the human condition. In the UK, the psychologist Eleanor Longden challenged the labels of mental health and schizophrenia, and in an interview she said that the voices in her head were a direct response to trauma earlier in her life and later they became benevolent and turned into guides (2015).

Potential effect of narrow interpretations

What happens when there is a narrow interpretation? When certain groups feel they are treated unfairly by society, they tend to become insular, cut themselves off and even work against that society. However, where cultures do not feel under threat, dialogue is possible.

Where cultures perceive themselves as oppressed, dialogue and communication can be very difficult. Fundamentalism encourages an 'us and them' mentality and it tends to flourish wherever a community feels threatened; members may not be interested in argument or debate and appear to be secure in their own truth.

There are several ways to address cultural sensitivity. In countries that have multicultural populations, ways forward for the health services might be to identify and support ways carers and clients prefer to interact with services – to learn about different communities, discuss their cultural knowledge and work closely with carers to ensure they understand healthcare options and how to support patient choices. Collaborative practice is most appropriate when working with others to provide a safe environment for patients to address any perceived unequal power relationships and conflicts.

How else might we integrate knowledge about faith and culture, in addition to popular understandings? How might we support change?

It is one thing to be familiar with knowledge at an academic or scholarly level but we need to integrate this knowledge with support for social change at the frontline.

There is often a time lag between acceptance and integration which may require changes in organizational structures and training. Sometimes organizations appear to be established as if to resist change and so innovations take time to be accepted. However, how might we take practical action ourselves to raise awareness within mainstream education?

ACADEMIC CONSENSUS ON TERMS AND PHENOMENOLOGY

There is a key problem when people from different cultures have 'anomalous' experiences and suggest these experiences offer insight into reincarnation, spirit possession or shamanic openings or awakenings. The problem arises when the same experiences are interpreted in many ways, negatively or positively, by different professions. For example, depending on context, some psychiatrists may identify auditory or visual experiences as indicative of pathology or schizophrenia. Some modern popular writers also distinguish between the two.

My proposition is that the same phenomena are interpreted differently according to different academic departments.

Would it have a beneficial effect on social wellbeing if scholars within different disciplines collaborated to raise awareness about the similarities of the nature of human experience? A dilemma exists in the field of mental health, where academics of different disciplines do not collaborate on 'extreme' or 'anomalous' human experience. Examples of this lack of communication between university departments can be seen below.

The disciplines mentioned below all study anomalous human experiences. However, the beliefs of individual scholars have influenced how extreme experiences and mental health have been regarded.

Religious studies departments at universities have conducted research with people who have had spontaneous religious and spiritual experiences. Transcendence, altered states of consciousness and out-of-body experiences were studied in transpersonal psychology, whereas paranormal psychology students researched clairvoyance, telepathy, mediumship and precognition.

Anomalous events such as near-death, end-of-life and out-of-body experiences have attracted the attention of psychiatrists, cardiologists and psychologists. Although transcultural psychiatry covered social and cultural interpretation of conditions and symptoms, it usually reframed them within a medical context. Medical anthropologists explore global beliefs about mental health, shamanic practices and spiritist aspects (the belief in spirits, spirit possession).

In addition to those mentioned above, some specialists have deliberately attempted to have experiences. These were first mentioned in Chapter 14. Practitioners who intended to achieve altered states of consciousness included clairvoyants and mediums who spoke with the deceased and shamans who claimed to actively engage with spirits.

Over time, certain practitioners in the west have remained silent about their visionary or auditory experiences (they were aware of the old assumption that their experiences were suggestive of mental ill health). Today, in closed online groups, people speak openly both about their experiences of and their anger towards their encounters with the mental health system.

In the previous chapter, we heard about the rise in mental health service users who were angry about medication and spoke out online against the psychiatric system. People who have had anomalous experiences claimed they were part of a spiritual emergency which resulted in profound personal transformation. They were joined by critical psychiatrists and other researchers who regarded extreme experiences as a way of spiritually breaking through to healing.

I mentioned the problem earlier in that same chapter of new students in medical schools and universities being repeatedly trained in old ways of thinking about anomalous phenomena. This was unfortunate in the case of those who had suffered from extreme experiences, as there was no consistency in how experiences were addressed. It was difficult to engage in a discussion about spiritual emergency, when professionals in allied disciplines insisted that the phenomena they researched were categorically different from the phenomena experienced during mental distress or extreme crisis.

It would be a small step for humankind for scholars to see the connection and raise awareness of experiences that are interpreted differently in different disciplines. It would be good to explore common ground in order to normalize experiences. The more people learn about other spontaneous altered states of consciousness and the deliberate experiences of specialist practitioners, the more it would benefit the dialogue around mental health.

ONE THEORY OF CHANGE

The Black Swan theory was developed by the American-Lebanese scholar, Nassim Nicholas Taleb (2010); he discussed the impact of transformational events which may be unpredictable and have a huge impact on society. In the aftermath of such events, people rationalized an explanation for it and its effects. In medieval times, people assumed there was no such creature as a black swan but now ornithologists know they are a normal species of water bird.

I wonder whether a black swan event is floating towards us on the horizon? Sometimes, even frequently, there seems to be a dissonance between mainstream television and social media; one presents certain types of news to consumers while the other presents data on the same news but interprets it differently.

In the UK for example, the mainstream BBC television service presented *In the Mind*, a series about mental health, and this prompted an immediate backlash from professionals and service users who claimed it misrepresented the scientific evidence. They asked the BBC to rectify its stance by presenting new perspectives.

I once heard about Procrustes, a rogue in ancient Greek mythology, who forced visitors to fit his iron bed. Are we (society) forcing people who have extreme experiences into an unnatural mould or are there other more compassionate strategies?

Within mental health, the evidence and research suggest there might be a huge shift coming. Some people who have had visionary or auditory experiences might assume they are accurate, that they were seeing what was really there. But what does this mean? Do some people believe apparitions and ghosts are real and that the spirits of the dead really exist? Do they believe they influence people's mental health and physical wellbeing?

These beliefs are so familiar to so many people in different cultures throughout the world. Are the anecdotes and personal narratives collected by anthropologists subjective? Are they part of a delusional ontology of the universe? Or are they correct and veridical? There is no longer a single truth, except to practise cultural humility, to observe and respond without judgement.

TOWARDS A WAY FORWARD
Further changes

Was it the ancient Greek philosopher Socrates who said the secret of change is to focus all of your energy, not on fighting the old, but on building the new? This seems to be happening. Recent years have seen the launch of books which question the status quo. These include my own *Spiritual Psychiatries* based on research in India (2014), Russell Razzaque's *Breaking Down is Waking Up* (2014), Katie Mottram's *Mend the Gap* (2014), James Davies' book *Cracked* (2013) and Robert Whitaker's *Anatomy of an Epidemic* (2010).

These were new times, involving reaching out for further support and collaboration. These included the Spiritual Crisis Network, the International Spiritual Emergence Network (ISEN) and the New Paradigm Alliance on Revisioning Mental Health. In 2015 a conference was held at Mundesley hospital in Norfolk entitled Evolving the New Paradigm: The Spirituality and Mental Health Breakthough. Speakers presented new ways of addressing spiritual emergencies using holistic strategies. Also there were Integrative Mental Health for You (IMHU) webinars in the USA which offered spiritist healing practices and personal empowerment.

That year there were conferences in London and Melbourne, Australia which aimed to revise a way to care for people who had extreme experiences. Participants included mental health nurses, carers, service users, practitioners, educators, managers and commissioners.

It seemed as if the tipping point had gone over towards change and change seemed to be moving swiftly. However, as I mentioned earlier, those responsible for mainstream education and training new students appeared less willing to teach towards a new paradigm.

Physicians already U-turning

I am aware that there appear to be two separate tracks; some social media sites represent what has been called New Age ways of thinking, then there is mainstream media, represented by television and the press. They do not necessarily appear to run along the same tracks or talk about the same issues.

In addition to the people and organizations mentioned above, below I will present a few examples of those striving towards combined collaborative change. There are groups which mediate the two tracks, like the discussion group set up by Chris Manning, a UK GP who experienced depression. He had treated patients for 'downstream' conditions and wanted to address 'upstream' health (2013).

Today, Manning explores strategies which reduce GP burnout and is interested in 'whole person' medicine at the College of Medicine (2012). Physicians are becoming increasingly concerned that they are suffering from the effects of witnessing and participating in traumatic events. They too are experiencing emotional distress and some feel that they have not been taught the consequences of practising medicine (Bailony 2015). There are projects by NHS England to offer GPs mental health support and the *British Journal of General Practice* (Van Gorden *et al.* 2016) is discussing Buddhist mindfulness techniques.

Research claims are currently being made by the Irish physician and psychotherapist, Terry Lynch. He disputes the biological origin of psychosis:

> The world is engulfed in a mass delusion regarding depression. The widespread belief that brain chemical imbalances are present in depression has no scientific basis. In fact, this is a fixed belief that meets all the criteria of a mass delusion. The brain chemical imbalance delusion has dominated medical, psychological and public thinking about depression for the past fifty years. (Lynch 2015, p.1)

The above quote by Terry Lynch was selected by the American psychologist, Phil Hickey, in his book review for *MadinAmerica* (Hickey 2015). MadinAmerica.com is a resource which gathers critical information on other ways of thinking about mental health. Some GPs were put off by the anti-psychiatry tone of Lynch's book, while other psychiatrists suggested techniques like Eye Movement Desensitization and Reprocessing (EMDR) were appropriate to address episodes of psychosis (Miller 2015).

At the Royal College of Psychiatry, there is a special interest group on spirituality and psychiatry and they have good archival resources on relevant publications. Nicki Crowley was a psychiatrist member interested in complementary therapies who had participated in the report (2006) *Putting the Soul Back into Psychiatry*. In her essay on psychosis and spirituality, she notes that psychosis is defined as 'any one of several altered states of consciousness, transient or persistent, that prevent integration of sensory or extrasensory information into reality models accepted by the broad consensus of society, and that lead to maladaptive behaviour and social sanctions' (1994).

With regard to spiritual emergency, Crowley has suggested:

> Observation from many disciplines, including clinical and experimental psychiatry, modern consciousness research, experiential psychotherapies, anthropological field studies, parapsychology, thanatology, comparative religions and mythology have contributed to the concept of 'spiritual emergency' a term that suggests both a crisis and an opportunity of rising to a new level of awareness or 'spiritual emergence'.

Her essay with its recommendations about ways to address spiritual emergency was written in 2006. I wonder to what extent it has become a normal part of medical education for trainee psychiatrists.

The 'paranormal' experiences Crowley mentioned could be linked with what participants talked about on the website Shades of Awakening.[1] I wrote an article on unusual experiences for MadinAmerica, Human Experiences in Academic Boxes (Tobert 2015b), because I thought it was necessary to draw in the links so society would stop making such experiences pathological. In this book, I have gathered narratives from different societies across the world to illustrate how they have understood the body, soul and spirit.

CHANGING CONSENSUS ON HUMAN EXPERIENCES

Psychosis appears to occur when an individual has a reduced ability to limit the content of their consciousness, an enhanced sensitivity and feels 'skinless' as if their body were permeable or without boundaries. It is unclear why some people have negative experiences whereas others have positive ones. Factors that predispose an individual towards mental illness could include their life events and circumstances, relationships, their spiritual or domestic environment or their underlying genetic pathology (depending on our respective belief systems). Perhaps certain people who experience psychosis may be slipping into a non-physical dimension and picking up material and confusing it with common consensus reality?

---

1   www.shadesofawakening.com, accessed 11/04/2016

What is the consensus regarding consciousness beyond death? What are our beliefs about what happens after death? Do we believe there is any afterlife or any kind of existence after death? When a person dies, does their consciousness die with them? To what extent do we believe human consciousness can exist without a body? And why is any of this significant to those who experience anomalous experiences and those who engage with people who have extreme experiences?

In western society, is it perhaps because we have a restricted ontological model for life after death that we experience some confusion when trying to understand topics such as psychosis, apparitions, near-death experiences and a lack of fear of death? Although we are beginning to accept the idea of consciousness after death, we may still find it problematic to embrace the concept of non-corporeal discarnate entities with personality (spirits).

Likewise, there has been reluctance to perceive that the human body is in some way porous and, like a radio transmitter, can change frequency, tune into different time and space frameworks or be tuned into by non-corporeal entities. Stemming from our denial of consciousness continuing after bodily death and our lack of understanding of the non-physical aspects of humans, perhaps we have developed our own culture-bound explanations for certain symptoms of mental suffering, perceptions of non-incarnate beings and memories from beyond the grave.

Consciousness and the paranormal

We used to assume that the key component of existence was matter – material things. Today we assume the universe is made up of energy and that our physical world and consciousness are intertwined. Marylyn Schlitz at the Institute of Noetic Studies has noted that the beliefs of an observer can influence the results of research (Schlitz et al. 2006).

Research into the manipulation of matter was carried out by Princeton University and the Institute of Noetic Sciences: their evidence invited us to ask about the nature of consciousness and its influence over matter. The CIA and Stanford University carried out research into remote viewing and a person's ability to project their awareness from one place to a distant location.

SUMMARY

In this chapter I have discussed why society needs to deepen its grasp of cultural understanding. I also noted that the interpretations of the UK Equality Act appear to have become rather narrow, if not in word, then in practice.

I have explored academic consensus on identifying the phenomenology of unusual or anomalous experiences. I also presented the Black Swan theory of change, where people rationalized an event after it occurred. The research evidence about anomalies and paranormal experience there but perhaps we deny its existence and continue regardless. In the field of mental health, it is of critical importance that we bridge the paradigms for the sake of social benefit. In the next chapter I will acknowledge the dilemmas we face and explore ways of addressing dissonance.

16

ACKNOWLEDGING DISSONANCE AS A WAY FORWARD

Truth about human experiences appears to be culture bound,
time specific, moveable and dependent on social consensus.

The previous chapter acknowledged the dissonance between mainstream academic studies and social media: the first presented certain types of data about human experiences to observers, while the second presented data on the same experiences but interpreted it differently. This dissonance is central to understanding the dilemma surrounding the ways we address mental health and acknowledging it is key to moving forwards. Figure 16.1 illustrates the dissonance between mainstream academia and popular social media. It points out that evidence from science is itself part of the tipping point of change, which leads to new ways of thinking.

I would like to identify the dissonance and key competing narratives in this chapter. I will start with a brief look at critical psychiatry, anti-psychiatry and the social meaning of symptoms. I then look at the triggers of distress.

The aim of this chapter is to present ways that the tipping point for change has already been reached. I will present the evidence of people who question biological factors which are proposed as part of diagnosis. I also lay out material which illustrates waves of change: evidence from professionals who consider medication is harmful and who want to see change swiftly occurring.

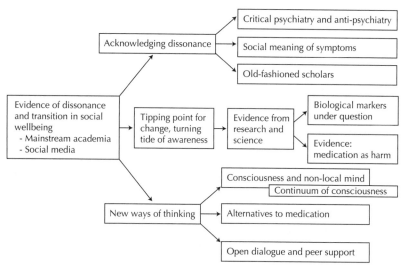

Figure 16.1. Dissonance and Transition

New ways of thinking are presented, ones which have gained currency in terms of consciousness, the non-local mind and parapsychology. I present suggestions for a series of alternative therapeutic strategies for social health and wellbeing. These are alternatives to pharmaceuticals and include Open Dialogue and peer support. It is by acknowledging this dissonance of beliefs that we can find a way forward towards positive change.

ACKNOWLEDGING DISSONANCE

Recently a number of researchers and practitioners have come out directly against psychiatry and mental health treatment. For example, the Australian psychiatrist Niall McLaren has questioned the basic principles of his profession (2013).

Others have questioned the new addition to the DSM-IV on freethinking and nonconformity (oppositional defiant disorder). The psychiatric term 'anosognosia' (not being able to recognize you have an illness) has been mocked. It has been used for those with Alzheimer's disease who do not have insight into the illness. Some researchers have questioned scientific evidence about markers in the brain and the effectiveness of medication.

Critical psychiatry

Joanna Moncrieff is a British psychiatrist and critic of the current biomedical model of mental disorders. Together with other psychiatrists, she is sceptical of the belief about brain diseases and their required pharmaceutical treatments. She often speaks about the medicalization of distress and how this neutralizes a person's own understanding of meaning. She writes:

> We will likely never be able to fully account for why some people experience extreme mental states, but we know that poverty, unemployment, insecure attachments, familial disruption, low self-esteem, abuse, etc. play a role for many. We would be better concentrating on how to eliminate these from our society if we really want to reduce the impact of mental disorder, rather that pouring more money into the bottomless pit of genetic research. (Moncrieff 2014)

Moncrieff has come out claiming that psychiatry actually causes harm, which of course was widely denied, and she said she had become sad about her profession. She has questioned the traditional assumptions that psychiatric drugs targeted underlying diseases and has suggested it was fraudulent to say they corrected chemical imbalances. She suggests we examine the real nature of drugs to practise better psychiatry (2009).

There were other professionals who shared her thoughts on pharmaceuticals and their inquiry resulted in 2015 in the Maudsley Debate exploring the topic of medication and harm. They asked whether we had reached a turning point:

> For the last 30 years those of us critical of the overprescribing and harms of psychiatric medications have been on the losing side, in the face of a powerful industry-backed medical model that has crowded out alternative voices and visions. The real importance of Wednesday's Maudsley Debate is that it symbolized what the critical community has been sensing for some time now – that the tide is finally turning. (CEP 2015)

Practitioners were explicit that scientific research evidence was not providing the required data. An Australian-based survey was carried out to determine the prevalence and correlates of mental disorders in households from 18 countries throughout the world, which included

31,261 adults. The conclusions of the research suggested that the epidemiologic features of psychotic episodes were 'more nuanced than previously thought' (McGrath *et al.* 2015) – in other words, not clearly identifiable.

The British psychiatrist, Phil Thomas, in his review of Scull's book (2015) on *Madness and Civilization*, which offered a history of western world psychiatry, wrote: 'our primary responsibility is to see the mad person not as an other but as ourselves. Only then may it be possible to break free of the tragic wheel of misfortune with which we have bound the mad and ourselves over the last 250 years' (Thomas 2015). Thomas was one of the founder members of the Critical Psychiatry Network.

Anti-psychiatry

Psychiatry has been accused of not being a legitimate branch of medicine and people have considered it as having been used to police 'socially unacceptable behaviour'. The term anti-psychiatry started to be used in 1960s when the loudest critics were psychiatrists themselves. They questioned the medicalization of mental ill health, the existence of mental illness, the power to detain individuals and the repression of the human spirit, saying psychiatric hospitals were more like prisons. They reminded us of cases in Nazi Germany and in Russia where psychiatrists were the forceful arm of oppressive regimes: people who were considered politically or morally deviant could be controlled.

The Citizens Commission on Human Rights (CCHR) was established in 1969 by the Church of Scientology and the psychiatrist Thomas Szasz, who wrote *The Myth of Mental Illness* (2010). The CCHR gathered stories about the inappropriate behaviour of psychiatrists and ran publicity campaigns advertising misuse. It started when patients were being stripped of their human rights; they wanted to eradicate abuse and advocated alternatives to pharmaceutical treatments.

The CCHR's mission statement was: 'To eradicate psychiatric abuse and brutality in the field of mental health, bringing about safety and security for those suffering any degree of mental problems'. When staff there heard I was doing research in the area of mental health, they gave me a free copy of their compendium: a reference book of psychiatry's destructive practices.

SOCIAL MEANING OF SYMPTOMS

Why are social meaning and context so important? The psychiatrist, Viktor Frankl has suggested that 'meaning in life' was more important for humans rather than happiness. He emphasized the importance of hope for human wellbeing (2008).

However, during World Mental Health Week in the UK, an article in *The Guardian* illustrated the crises in mental health services, where people who used the services felt there was no hope. We learnt that two-thirds of the people who had depression received no treatment (Topping 2014).

Thomas was aware of the dilemmas facing his profession of psychiatry and the UK mental health services (2014). He emphasized the importance of context in understanding distress, in understanding a person's cultural, historical and social influences which gave meaning to their lives. He suggested psychiatrists should move away from the biological origins of distress and its pharmacological treatments.

The British psychologist, Mary Boyle (2015), has also discussed the importance of acknowledging context as a cause of mental distress while speaking at the Division of Clinical Psychology's annual conference in Glasgow. She spoke about the professional avoidance of evidence about social and material context, asking whether clinical psychologists were fearful of social context. In a similar vein, the results of some research correlating depression and suicide with unemployment and poverty were kept concealed in America (Levine 2015a).

At the same time, in India, some private psychiatrists appeared to be forging a way ahead in their thinking about the triggers of distress, incorporating spiritual as well as social factors. Those who practised integral health suggested that counselling might be enhanced if practitioners considered a range of inner and outer triggers of disharmony (Basu 2015).

Old-fashioned scholars

When I facilitated training seminars for staff, I discovered frontline medical and healthcare staff were themselves willing to consider and start using new therapeutic strategies. However, the problem lay more profoundly with the medical and healthcare education system.

Although change is the only constant in life, some academic scholars rigidly maintained the educational classification systems that they had been taught and with which they were familiar. For example, when I taught medical students about cultural diversity and the wide-ranging variety of triggers of mental distress, students repeated verbatim what they had been taught the day before by their more old-fashioned educators who adhered to narrow biomedical models.

This is a problem as new students are currently being trained in old ways of thinking about anomalous phenomena. They are taught that this or that ethnic group has a propensity towards psychosis, without considering a person's historical background. This is particularly unfortunate in the case of those who suffer from extreme experiences, breakdowns or spiritual emergencies.

When professionals believed in the diseases of the brain model of psychosis, then it followed that they assumed pharmaceutics needed to be used to address the chemical imbalance of the brain. In that way, myth followed myth. I will explore the evidence from science which supports the need for change below.

TIPPING POINT FOR CHANGE
Evidence from research and science

It seems that the tipping point for radical change is fast approaching. The journalist, Antony Funnell, has claimed some psychiatrists were divided on whether to stop using the DSM: 'there's a growing rift within the field of psychiatry over the effectiveness of traditional mental health treatment, with some practitioners declaring it's time to throw out the diagnostic handbook and start again from scratch' (Funnell 2014).

Perhaps the tipping point has even been reached and has been surpassed. The tide has turned. In London, there was an amazing one-day conference on critical psychiatry which explored the harm done by the over-prescription of medication (CEP 2015). The first speaker was the social anthropologist, James Davies, who had interviewed the originators of the DSM about how it first came into being.

Davies learnt there was no scientific evidence behind the definitions of symptoms (2014). His controversial book, *Cracked*, illustrated how scientific research was manipulated to benefit pharmaceutical pockets without reference to scientific evidence. He described how psychiatric drugs were supported by mass marketing and set out the human cost of pathologizing suffering.

Bob Whitaker also spoke at that conference. He presented data on corruption and bad institutions: on the economies which influenced good individuals in the practice of diagnosis, research and treatment (2015). Another ardent critical voice was that of psychologist Professor John Read. He commented on the nature of illness as it is marketed in the press, asking on social media: 'How can we address the causes of human misery if we don't get rid of this drug company maintained delusion?'.

There appeared to be a mismatch between the discontent of critical psychiatrists, the rage felt by those who were anti-psychiatry and those psychiatrists/educators who taught students in medical schools. There was a mismatch between the mainstream media and social media. I was shocked to discover that students were still being taught about the propensity of particular ethnic groups towards psychosis, an opinion which was racist and completely disregarded people's histories of oppression, repression and suppression. The assumed biological markers of mental illness were being presented and the lack of evidence denied.

Biological markers under question

In 2009, the Dutch psychiatrist Jim van Os proposed abolishing the diagnosis of schizophrenia due to the lack of validity and the risk of 'fundamental attribution error' associated with the label (van Os and Kapur 2009). The disease model of mental health was also profoundly questioned by clinical psychologist, Peter Kinderman (2014). A recent review researched by an American doctoral student presented the history of the chemical imbalance hypothesis for mental ill health and the evidence base for it (Schultz 2015).

Other psychiatrists also spoke out; in the USA, Robert Berezin commented on 'biological markers' or the lack of them for psychosis (2015a). The key issues around diagnosis came to a crisis point and it seemed to depend on the personal belief system of the practitioner as to whether they believed in a recovery model or a diseases of the brain model of mental health (Karter 2015).

Jonathan Metzl was professor of sociology and psychiatry and his research was key in questioning the disease-oriented interpretation of psychosis (2010). He became aware that the hospital where he worked tended to diagnose African Americans with schizophrenia because of their ideas about civil rights. He said 'I focus on ways published case studies explicitly connected clinical presentations of African American men with the politics of the civil rights movement in ways that treated aspirations for liberation and civil rights as symptoms of mental illness' (Metzl 2014). Phil Thomas (2014) had earlier stressed the need to consider adversity, oppression and abuse.

In the past, western-biased intelligence tests carried out by psychologists and psychiatrists on indigenous First Nation American people 'proved they were inferior'. Today we recognize 'historical trauma' some of the time. The American psychologist Walker reported on the high suicide rate amongst those First Peoples who had been oppressed and the women coerced into sterilization (2015).

In Australia, tens of thousands of Aboriginal people were admitted to hospitals with self-harm (Georgatos 2015). One woman, Gayili Yunupingu, used community strategies to reduce suicide among her people: art and craftwork were key practices towards healing. She offered caring in a culturally sensitive manner and invited people to tell their stories and explore their pain (Margetts 2015). This appears to be an Open Dialogue strategy in origin.

Peter Kinderman, professor of clinical psychology at the University of Liverpool, argued that biological factors were far less important than social factors in people's lives and that our medical bias wrongly convinced us that medication was the answer. He has suggested it is time to re-evaluate our explanatory models for depression (Belger 2014).

Similarly in Ireland, research claims have been made by Terry Lynch, a physician and psychotherapist, who disputed the biological origin of psychosis (2015). On the myth of chemical imbalance, the US activist Sera Davidow (2015) has claimed that '*many* psychiatrists have stepped up and acknowledged that there is no identifiable chemical imbalance to which they can point, and researchers have concurred'. Where do we go from here?

Evidence: medication as harm

New research has investigated the ways in which funding by drug companies has corrupted psychiatric practice over the last few decades. Robert Whitaker and Lisa Cosgrove have documented challenges to the biological origin of mental disorders, recorded concerns about informed consent for psychiatric drugs and the profession's practice of creating pathology out of normal behaviour (2015).

The authors investigated how pharmaceutical money had corrupted the American Psychiatric Association during the past 35 years. They documented how the psychiatric establishment misled the American public about the biology of mental disorders, the validity of psychiatric diagnoses and the safety and efficacy of its drugs. They asked whether psychiatric drugs fix 'chemical imbalances' in the brain or whether they actually *created imbalances*.

One of the authors, Robert Whitaker, said during an interview:

> The assumption is that individuals within the institution can't see that their behaviour has been corrupted by 'economies of influence'. And so, when those outside the institution begin pointing out the corruption in it, those within it may construct a narrative that protects their self-image. In this case, psychiatrists need to protect their image as honest researchers and as physicians who put the interests of their patients first.

Furthermore, he asked for all scientific trials on the beneficial effects of psychiatric medication to be made available (2015).

The research evidence base has been questioned. There have also been cover-ups of the negative side effects suggested by pharmaceutical data and adverse drug reactions have been hidden. Some researchers have suggested corruption was at play, as Bruce Levine (2015b) discovered when he interviewed the authors of *Psychiatry under the Influence*.

The Danish physician, Peter Gøtzsche, has explained why he thought antidepressants caused more harm than good (2014) and he mentioned the problems with pharmaceuticals saying they had too many side effects, likening them to organized crime. Multiple claims have surfaced that psychiatric medication is both harmful and dangerous.

The psychiatrist, Robert Berezin, who taught at Harvard Medical School has claimed that pharmaceuticals were destructive and that there was plenty of evidence for this. He suggested that '[p]sychiatry is fast approaching a death spiral which we as a society may not be able to recover from' (2015b).

Word has gone out from the New York psychiatrist, Peter Breggin, who has expressed a desire to reform the system, that patients should be careful: 'Psychiatric drugs including antidepressants, benzodiazepines, stimulants can cause manic psychosis and other conditions resulting in suicide, violence or criminal behaviors such as shoplifting, robbery and more' (2009). He also spoke out against psychiatric drugs for children and the lack of evidence for their effectiveness and the harm they may cause. Professionals seemed to be turning against their old practices of diagnosis and treatment.

NEW WAYS OF THINKING
Consciousness and non-local mind

In what additional ways might we interpret symptoms of distress? How appropriate might it be today to explore psychiatric and shamanic practices together? Some years ago I compared the roles of diagnosis and treatment within shamanism and psychiatry. I explored their methods of working and their function to alleviate human suffering and maintain social order. Shamanic practice was focused on an individual within society and the environment, whereas early psychiatry had been focused on an individual's mind/brain. In each case their diagnoses were linked to their own explanatory models of causation (Tobert 2015a).

Brodie (2015) has suggested that shamans and psychics tune into some kind of non-local realm to access information. It may be the same realm that people experiencing anomalous experiences tap into unbidden and spontaneously – they may then experience that they are not sure where they are, as it doesn't fit with their current frameworks of understanding.

Thanks to social media, people have become more explicit about their experiences and how they interpreted them, including one case of extreme clairvoyance, where a woman set out her own experiences. Such experiences may also be claimed by clairvoyants, psychics and shamans who can control them and have a framework to understand them. Some human beings appeared to be permeable and susceptible to outside influences. Of course, these experiences may be interpreted differently, depending on the reader's own beliefs.

The American psychiatrist, Michael Miovic (2009), who spent time in India exploring consciousness by way of the writings of the sage/philosopher, Sri Aurobindo, explained:

It is becoming always clearer that not only does the capacity of our total consciousness far exceed that of our organs, the senses, the nerves, the brain, but that even for our ordinary thought and consciousness these organs are only their habitual instruments and not their generators. Consciousness uses the brain which its upward strivings have produced, [the] brain has not produced nor does it use the consciousness.

In his conclusion, Miovic wrote: 'The existence of soul and Spirit as realities independent of matter has not yet been experimentally verified – and may never be.' His colleague, the integral psychiatrist Soumitra Basu wrote on the cultivation of faith (2000). His support was instrumental in my research for *Spiritual Psychiatries* (Tobert 2014).

Continuum of consciousness

Psychosis and spiritual awakening appear to be part of the same process. There is a relationship between paranormal experience, religious experience and the symptoms of schizophrenia; the phenomena appear to lie on the extreme ends of a continuum.

In the past, I used to start conversations with colleagues in different academic disciplines about mental health or spiritual crisis. I found several colleagues who thought their discipline covered experiential human phenomena which had nothing to do with mental health.

It was difficult to progress in an argument about spiritual emergency if professionals in allied disciplines insisted the phenomena they researched were categorically different from the phenomena experienced during mental distress or extreme crisis.

These differences of opinion meant there was no consistency in the way such experiences were scientifically explored. It appeared to be a fairly small step to see the connection and raise awareness of experiences that are interpreted differently in different disciplines in different countries. If only we could explore common ground, it would benefit the global dialogue about mental health.

If each discipline were willing to learn more about other states of consciousness and the phenomena of specialist practitioners like psychics or shamans, it would help. I have written an article inviting educators in different disciplines to sit around the same table and discuss anomalous experiences and mental wellbeing (Tobert 2015b).

Whilst writing this section, I received a Skype call from Switzerland, from two people who were professionally interested in communication from beyond death. After I gave a talk there, participants in the group realized people with 'psychosis' may be receiving data from other worlds, which is what they were interested in and wanted to chat with me about. The willingness to change is well underway.

The essay by Dr Nicki Crowley (2006) on spiritual emergence and the need to incorporate training on spirituality was awarded a prize by the Spirituality and Psychiatry Special Interest Group of the Royal College of Psychiatrists. In addition to such prizes, we need to ensure that the education system in medical schools is modified so that students are taught new ways of thinking about mental health and not the recycled racist packages of former years.

It seems as if there is a fast opening into altered states of consciousness, with so many people in the last few decades having extreme experiences, data overload and amplified sensations. Psychiatrists like Stan Grof (1989) interpreted these fast awakenings as spiritual emergencies before others and the clinical psychologist, Isabel Clarke, realized psychosis and spirituality were on a continuum (2001).

ALTERNATIVES TO MEDICATION

One ancient way to address suffering consisted of Deep Listening, mentioned by the Vietnamese Buddhist monk, Thich Nhat Hanh (1999, 2014). Perhaps his philosophy including mindfulness is what those being trained in Open Dialogue are being taught? In London, change is swiftly underway and a research post has been created to explore alternative strategies like Open Dialogue for efficacy. Based within a psychiatry department, the project is headed by the critical psychiatrist Joanna Moncrieff. Results may change the way people diagnosed with schizophrenia and psychosis are treated.

Along a similar line in Europe, Compassion Focused Therapy (CFT) has been researched. It was tested on 40 adults with 'schizophrenia-spectrum disorder' and the intervention was found to promote greater clinical improvement and emotional recovery from psychosis (Braehler et al. 2013).

In America, the winds of change are already blowing from Big Sur in California. Michael Cornwall is a psychotherapist who experienced an extreme state without medication or treatment. Today he specializes in offering psychotherapy for people in extreme psychotic states in community settings and sanctuaries where medications are not used.

Perhaps the collaborative training offered by Cornwall and Lukoff could be embedded as part of core educational curricula for frontline practitioners elsewhere in the world. They have set out ways of compassionately responding to people in extreme states. Their aim was for people struggling with madness to explore their emotions of distress in a supportive sanctuary. The idea of Soteria (the Greek goddess of safety and deliverance from harm) as a sanctuary also came from California and was replicated in Europe and Australia.

In America, the National Institutes of Health reported on positive evidence for team-based treatment strategies for first episodes of psychosis. John Kane, the head of their early treatment project, said:

> The goal is to link someone experiencing first episode psychosis with a coordinated specialty care team as soon as possible after psychotic symptoms begin… Our study shows that this kind of treatment can be implemented in clinics around the country. It improves outcomes and the effects are greater for those with a shorter duration of untreated psychosis. (NIH 2015)

In the USA Dion Zessin (2015), a researcher into alternative strategies for addressing psychiatric distress, has gathered evidence-based alternatives to psychiatric drugs called the *Codex Alternus*. It is a reference book for practitioners and carers and includes Ayurvedic, African and Chinese remedies, as well as practices of exercise and mindfulness and creative therapies. However, it retains the psychiatric diagnostic labels of schizophrenia, bipolar and so forth.

Peer support

In New York, the Parachute Project has made peer support integral to the delivery of services. After a long time on the borders of therapeutic activity, peer support for those who have had experiences has appeared to take centre stage at some places. This is both to support sufferers and to train frontline staff from statutory organizations: 'Participants viewed peer support as especially valuable because of the opportunity for a non-treatment based, normalizing relationship' (Gidugu *et al.* 2014).

Statutory practitioners were aware of the importance of working with peers because they had inner strength from lived experience and they could participate as co-therapists. Peers felt that they changed the dynamics and the sense of hierarchy within the system; they had shared understandings with a sufferer and permitted a sense of hope for the future (Hendry *et al.* 2014).

Those who heard voices had learnt to talk back to them and national newspapers were reporting their stories more sensitively (Adams 2015). In 1988, a movement to support voice hearers was established, inspired by Professor Marius Romme and Sondra Escher. The movement was mobilized globally in 35 countries (Adams 2015, Romme and Escher 1993).

Professional people also started opening up with their own personal stories of transformation. Chris Manning spoke out about 'whole person medicine' and the Canadian physician, Angele Beaudoin, was interviewed about her own direct experience of the mental health system. New York practitioner Abdi Assadi spoke out on spiritual bypass and psychology and emphasized the need to engage with the therapeutic process rather than bypass our emotions.

London Conference on Open Dialogue

Open Dialogue as a strategy for treatment is mentioned in earlier chapters, to support those going through first episode psychosis. In Finland, Open Dialogue was not an alternative to psychiatric practice, it *was* the psychiatric service (Seikkula 2011, Seikkula *et al.* 2011). Changes in practice there reported that 75% of people experiencing psychosis returned to work or study within two years of an event and 20% were still on antipsychotic medication at their two-year follow-up.

Whilst writing this chapter, I attended an Open Dialogue conference in London. The meeting was attended by around 1000 people, service users, peer support workers, carers, complimentary practitioners and medical and healthcare staff.

Speakers informed the audience that the key practice was 'to accept others without condition'. The practice also allowed staff to have *agency*, so they felt they could work with a healing process, rather than the medication having agency.

One of the key questions that arose several times was how we might address psychiatrists' anxiety about the new system. The older strategy was to identify a label and reduce or remove symptoms, rather than reaching the meaning of symptoms. It was to avoid suffering, rather than be present with suffering.

Participants who attended the Peer-supported Open Dialogue courses experienced other dilemmas; they had learnt a new way of working but had to return to their former departments using 'normal' practice. The usual belief was a disease of the brain theory of causation, with medication to treat chemical imbalances. The psychiatrist, Russell Razzaque, argued for a whole system change across the NHS to support the research evidence of the effectiveness of this strategy.

There was a concern about colonizing other countries with this approach. The question about whether Open Dialogue was culturally applicable was put forward. However, I was aware that other cultures in Africa already practised a variant of this; the anthropologist Victor Turner has reported on public rituals to address personal suffering among the Ndembu (Turner 1967). In Somalia, Lewis (2002) has reported on the way spirits took over women and allowed them to speak their mind, in a way which would not have been culturally tolerated outside the ceremony.

In the above examples, personal suffering was presented in public drama, and healing did not take place until all secrets were spoken. One of the last comments at that event was from an African man, angry that he had been diagnosed with paranoid schizophrenia, which he claimed only happened because he was African. This served as a timely reminder to all present of the importance of cultural humility.

Participants at the conference considered that we needed to create a restorative justice or truth and reconciliation approach to address the needs of staff and previous patients. We needed to address the anxiety of psychiatric staff and the anger of former patients who had been treated according to the old system.

The next step was to deal with inequities: political, environmental, racist, those due to poverty and other triggers of distress that breached human rights. Is it enough to listen to a person's narrative of distress without addressing social and environmental causes of suppression?

17

TOWARDS POSITIVE CHANGE

Cultural U-turns on the changing nature of truth
appear to be ubiquitous and inevitable.

In this chapter I consider which strategies we might take towards positive change in mental health. In the previous chapter I mentioned organizations which are already practising what they preach and creating dynamic change, but here I will look at what the rest of us might do. What direct action might we take towards change? There has been a huge change in the services available to people experiencing distress but they are not ubiquitously available.

There is an awareness that one size does not fit all, that there is a plurality of ways of interpreting experience and that truth is culturally determined. There are completely different existential ways of understanding the world and reality. In this chapter I will look at ways of negotiating through these multiple interpretations of reality.

The first step is to acknowledge the dilemma, then explore a truth and reconciliation strategy with all stakeholders. An alliance of all the organizations standing up for change would be good. Then we need to change the system at its core so new practitioners are aware of the new thinking as part of their mainstream education. We need to lobby those in power to ensure positive change happens (see Figure 17.1, which illustrates a range of strategies towards change).

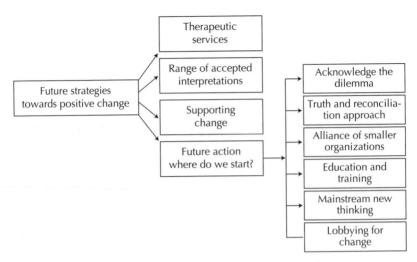

Figure 17.1. Future Strategies towards Positive Change

FUTURE STRATEGIES AND CHANGE
Therapeutic services

There has been a huge appetite to change mainstream services, to challenge them publicly, quickly, intellectually and rigorously. The old fear – that one would not get appropriate treatment unless one remained silent – appears to have vanished. An unstoppable wave of discontent is gaining momentum.

People are using evidence-based data to turn old thinking on its head. They question the old statistics and the way research data was selected for publication. They are producing evidence for the new therapeutic strategies and acting upon it. This is very important for the future wellbeing of society.

Therapeutic practices are thus changing for the better in some places. We all understand more about the triggers of distress. These are extremely positive changes. However, I still doubt whether the new practices are enough to address the complexities of different cultural beliefs about the origins of distress and the culturally relevant treatments. Also, I doubt that we have the popular media and most academic scholars with us. What would be ideal is universal understanding and change.

Range of accepted interpretations

Change is already happening. Invited by the Equality and Diversity Manager at an NHS trust, I facilitated seminars for consultant psychiatrists, medical doctors and frontline healthcare staff in the chapel room of a former psychiatric hospital. We explored cultural perceptions of human existence and compared cultural interpretations of symptoms of spirit possession and schizophrenia. We discussed a range of strategies for treatment and we explored the importance of spiritual beliefs about death and beyond for understanding extreme experiences. Participants agreed cultural humility was the way forward, negotiating with each client about their beliefs.

In earlier chapters, epigenetics was considered in relation to people's loss and trauma; it is the study of reactions which influence our human DNA. I also presented brief material on pre-natal experiences, those memories which appeared to occur to those who had experienced the Holocaust and people in other societies who had ancestral memories.

I then gave examples of Indian healing traditions, with examples from *Spiritual Psychiatries*, together with alternative healing remedies in India and the wisdom of the philosophers Sri Aurobindo and Sri Ramana Maharshi. I noted that the example set by some spiritual Indian psychiatrists appeared to illustrate more compassionate strategies for treatment and the belief in a recovery model. Changes in western psychiatry might benefit and be supported by evidence from some practices in the east.

In addition, I explored cultural interpretations of the symptoms of distress from Africa, Brazil and Siberia and compared these with shamanic traditions in various countries. Finally, I discussed experiences from a paranormal perspective and from those who studied religious experiences.

I would now like to present a selection of options for a way forward to address the dissonance between mainstream practice and spiritual awareness as presented on social media. My aspiration is that the competing narratives can be acknowledged and used as part of the negotiation towards change.

Supporting change

Where do we go from here? How can we acknowledge the dilemma and support those medical and healthcare staff who understand the need for change and want to or have to remain in working relationships with their peers?

Profound differences of opinion about consciousness and existential reality may occur between different staff within an organization which may result in anxiety and stress. Conflict may develop when individuals do not feel they are being heard. Silence may be an easier route, when career, income and respect from peers need to be preserved.

However, there may still be issues around inequalities, even innocently, when seminars are run. There may be academic inequalities: for example, in terms of who gets the jobs and whose work is published to maintain the status quo around 'real knowledge'. Who is asked to speak at conferences? Which peer or which scholar is invited to talk? Subtle change must occur to lift the old-fashioned systems of controlling knowledge.

In the UK, a new alliance is being established called ReVisioning Mental Health. It is a coalition of organizations and individuals who actively promote contemporary, person-centred mental healthcare. It is made up of service users, carers, clinicians and members of the public who are committed to promoting mental wellbeing for all. They want to address current struggles between the mental health system and service users. They are offering to collaborate with public, statutory and voluntary sector organizations to promote reconciliation.

In addition to this, the International Spiritual Emergency Network raise awareness of spiritual awakening.

The strategy for negotiation and dialogue used in Paris for the climate talks sounded like a useful, contemporary way to engage people with different opinions and could also be used for healing purposes. Known as *indaba*, the process is South African Zulu and is used to simplify discussions between many people; it allows everyone to voice their opinion in order to reach a consensus. Each stakeholder is encouraged to speak personally, state their threshold of need and suggest a solution suitable for the common purpose.

At this stage, I wonder what positive suggestions I might make – in light of the evidence – to support change and develop positive strategies for moving forward for social benefit.

I have been explicit about spiritual influences on mental health. I feel obliged to offer a series of potential solutions for discussion, to ways of understanding health, the body and human existence. I want to offer suggestions to collaborate with medical and health professionals and educators to maintain change for social wellbeing. But where do we start?

FUTURE ACTION
Acknowledge the dilemma

To begin with, we need to acknowledge there is a dilemma. If we evaluate the scientific evidence regarding the effectiveness of medication and certain other treatments like ECT, then the need for profound change is suggested.

If we acknowledge the evidence regarding the effectiveness of Open Dialogue training and Peer-supported Open Dialogue in particular, then we must develop a strategy for working with current practitioners; in the UK, some psychiatrists are doing sterling work towards change in the NHS.

Truth and reconciliation approach

Perhaps we need a truth and reconciliation approach to acknowledge the anger and distress of service users who experienced the former system. This would also address the anxiety of staff who are aware of new ways but who do not know how to get them into current practice in their health departments. We need a reconciliation service between professionals who were trained in Peer-supported Open Dialogue and those in the same department who may follow a more old-fashioned approach.

Alliance of smaller organizations

There needs to be an effective alliance of the plethora of smaller organizations who each appear to be working towards change, like ReVisioning Mental Health or ISEN, Soteria and the Hearing Voices Network (HVN).

The International Society for Psychological and Social Approaches to Psychosis (ISPS) started in Switzerland and has groups in 19 countries. It promotes a psychotherapeutical treatment approach for people experiencing psychosis. It was started in the 1950s by two Swiss psychiatrists who considered the treatment for schizophrenia was not appropriate. They sought a more humanistic approach.

Education and training

In the USA, cultural competency is already required as an essential part of core mainstream medical education. In the UK, online training about the Equality Act is an isolated, individual training course which does not require direct self-reflection or discussion with peers. However, within the UK's education system, every school currently has a duty to illustrate ways in which they comply with the Equalities Act on spiritual, moral, social and cultural wellbeing.

Systematic change is required within the education system. Cultural competency is now a requirement according to the new DSM-5 but cultural humility and equity are also needed: the ability to ask a sufferer about their beliefs and practices to effect healing. What happened, rather than what are your symptoms? With cultural humility, a practitioner need not learn everything about every society but would just need to find the time and space to ask the relevant questions. This is already taught as part of Open Dialogue training.

We must unpack the meaning of the term 'recovery', which for some means clinical recovery when the symptoms have gone whereas for others it means discovering a resilient life of hope where they are in control of their decisions.

Also essential is training which raises awareness of plural frameworks of health and theories of illness causation, communication strategies and self-reflection about the influence of personal belief systems. The training courses which I offer in medical schools and hospitals include information about new frameworks of knowledge and cultural frameworks of illness causation, including spiritual influences.

Students can be trained in the use of communication strategies to determine a patient's social and religious perspectives on the meaning of their illness, their gender and their personal history, as the current Peer-supported Open Dialogue does, but with more of an emphasis on cultural awareness. We need to raise awareness of the plurality of frameworks for understanding the body, health and self: life and death and beliefs about survival beyond death.

Mainstream new thinking

Mainstreaming training of medical students requires a complete change so they are no longer taught about the predispositions of this or that ethnic group or about chemical disorders of the brain which can only be healed by medication.

We need to offer certified courses, with post-registration training to those staff who are in post and want to be supported by other ways of thinking about mental ill health. Webinars could be made available so this material is accessible across the globe.

Post-registration education could be used to raise awareness of more sensitive data collection strategies about the way patient ethnicity and personal narratives are recorded, plus a deeper awareness of the social context of ethnicity and health. There is no room for subtle racist education about 'predispositions'.

Lobbying

Politicians and senior staff at the Department of Health must be lobbied about the new ways of thinking. Likewise, the deans of medical schools need to be aware of the change so that their staff can modify the medical school curricula. Inequalities need to be addressed.

Medical and healthcare educational leaders may welcome the following actions in order to make manifest a future vision for social inclusion. Collaboration with deans of education is essential so cultural awareness becomes a core part of the mainstream curriculum in medical schools and associated healthcare educational establishments.

We need to lobby government policy makers so they develop a central, online archive of academic and grey literature in the UK. In this way, local evaluation and research reports about effective strategies would not be lost in the grey mists of local authority office shelves. If this is not done, the only reports visible to the global public and professionals would be those accepted for peer review which may or may not adhere to the old-fashioned party line.

In addition to a central online archive, we need to develop a strategy for systematically evaluating recommendations from research and consultation and take appropriate action to make manifest reasonable change. This must include work from community evaluations, which is not necessarily published, but may offer useful insights at the frontline.

If this is not done, we (society) will tend to go into a feedback loop of repeating research and consultation without ever taking direct action towards change. Chris Argyris was a business theorist who claimed organizations took action to inhibit social change: they conducted cycles of research and consultation but took no action towards change.

It is now the time to take action based on scientific research and consultation. It is time for medical schools to address their teaching about extreme human experiences and spiritual awakening to incorporate the new knowledge. On a positive note, in collaboration with medical and health service educators, we can support the current changing medical paradigm around mental health.

There is room for another cultural U-turn on social and mental wellbeing. This would be in line with our normal practice, seen earlier in this book, of consistently making U-turns over time.

BIBLIOGRAPHY

Aaltonen, J. *et al.* (2011) "The comprehensive open-dialogue approach in western lapland: i. the incidence of non-affective psychosis and prodromal states". *Psychosis* 3:3, pp.179–91.

Adams, W.L. (2015) "The Enemy Within: People Who Hear Voices in Their Heads Are Being Encouraged to Talk Back". *Independent*, 25 January 2015.

Allix, S. and Bernstein, P. (eds) (2009) *Manuel clinique des expériences extraordinaires.* Paris: Institut de recherche sur les expériences extraordinaires.

Alvarado, C. (2014) "The Paranormal is (Still) Normal". Available at https://carlossalvarado.wordpress.com/2014/09/13/the-paranormal-is-still-normal/, accessed on 08 April 2016.

Alvarado, C. (2015) "Analyses of Healing Studies". Available at https://carlossalvarado.wordpress.com/2015/01/13/analyses-of-healing-studies/, accessed on 08 April 2016.

Assadi, A. (2015) "Spiritual Bypass". Available at http://abdiassadi.com/abdi-assadi-podcast-spiritual-bypass-2/, accessed on 08 April 2016.

Azuonye, I.O. (1997) "A difficult case: Diagnosis made by hallucinatory voices". *British Medical Journal* 315, p.1685.

Badham, P. (1997) "The Evidence from Psychical Research." In P. Edwards (ed.), *Immortality.* New York: Prometheus Books.

Bailony, A. (2015) "Nobody Teaches a Physician the Emotional Consequences of Medicine". Available at www.kevinmd.com/blog/2015/08/nobody-teaches-a-physician-the-emotional-consequences-of-medicine.html, accessed on 08 April 2016.

Bandyopadhyay, M. *et al.* (2003) "Loss of Face: Violence against Women in South Asia." In L. Manderson, and L.R. Bennett, (eds) Violence against Women in Asian Societies. London: Routledge.

Barbato, A. (1998) "Schizophrenia and Public Health". Available at www.who.int/mental_health/media/en/55.pdf, accessed 08 April 2016.

Basu, S. (2000) *Integral Health: A Conscious Approach to Health & Healing.* Kripa: Sri Aurobindo Ashram Publications.

Basu, S. (2015) "Dealing with harmony". *NAMAH: The Journal of Integral Health* 23:2.

Battaglia, D. (1990) *On the Bones of the Serpent: Person, Memory and Mortality in Sabarl Island Society*. Chicago: University of Chicago Press.

BBC (n.d.) 'Honour crimes'. *BBC ethics guide*. Available at www.bbc.co.uk/ethics/honourcrimes/crimesofhonour_2.shtml, accessed on 11 August 2016.

Beaudoin, A. (2015) "A Physician's Plea for Hope". Available at http://crazywisefilm.com/2015/02/18/angele-beaudoin-physicians-plea-hope, accessed on 08 April 2016.

Belger, T. (2014) "Mental Health, Drugs and Robin Williams: A Liverpool Professor's Take on Actor's Suicide". *Liverpool Echo*, 15 August 2014.

Bentall, R. *et al.* (2011) "From adversity to psychosis: pathways and mechanisms from specific adversities to specific symptoms". *Social Psychiatry and Psychiatric Epidemiology* 49:7, pp.1011–22.

Berezin, R. (2015a) "Enough is Enough Series: 2-Year-Olds on Anti-Psychotics and Biological Markers for Psychosis". Available at http://robertberezin.com/enough-is-enough-series-4-2-year-olds-on-anti-psychotics-and-biological-markers-for-psychosis, accessed 08 April 2016.

Berezin, R. (2015b) "The Alternative to Drugs. The Real Treatment for Human Suffering". Available at http://robertberezin.com/the-alternative-to-drugs-the-real-treatment-for-human-suffering, accessed on 08 April 2016.

Berlin, E. and Fowkes, W. (1983) "A teaching framework for cross-cultural health care". *Western Journal of Medicine* 139:6, pp.934–8.

Betty, D. (2009) *Survivors Add New Voices to Dark Chapter in Medical History*. Mental Health Media Archive. Available at http://studymore.org.uk/mp001122.htm, accessed on 12 August 2016.

Bhui, K. and Bhugra, D. (2002a) "Explanatory models for mental distress". *British Journal of Psychiatry* 181, pp.6–7.

Bhui, K. and Bhugra, D. (2002b) "Mental illness in Black and Asian ethnic minorities". *Advances in Psychiatric Treatment* 8, pp.26–33.

Biswas, S. (2012) "How India Treats its Women". BBC News, 20 December 2012.

Borges, P. (2015) "Tribal Approaches to Mental Health Treatment, Thrive 2020". Available at www.youtube.com/watch?v=oIkMHtjwlIU, accessed on 08 April 2016.

Bowie, F. (2002) *Alistair Hardy Religious Experience Research Centre*, Occasional Paper, May 2002.

Bowie, F. (2013) "Anthropology and the paranormal: Report on a symposium at the Esalen Institute". *Paranthropology* 4:4.

Boyle, M. (2015) "Is Clinical Psychology Fearful of Social Context?" Available at www.youtube.com/watch?v=Kt4JcTDPUoc, accessed on 08 April 2016.

Braehler, C. *et al.* (2013) "Exploring change processes in compassion-focused therapy in psychosis". *British Journal of Clinical Psychology* 52:2, pp.199–214.

Breggin, P. (2009) *Medication Madness: The Role of Psychiatric Drugs in Cases of Violence, Suicide, and Crime.* New York: St Martin's Press.

Brennan, Z. (2011) "Special Investigation: Inside the Migrant Maternity Ward Where the NHS is Struggling to Cope". Mail Online, 7 May 2011.

Brodie, E. (2015) "The Science Behind Shamanism – Non-locality". Available at www.thesacredscience.com/blog1/the-science-behind-shamanism-non-locality, accessed on 08 April 2016.

Brown, P.L. (2009) "A Doctor for Disease, a Shaman for the Soul". *New York Times,* 19 September 2009.

Capdecomme, M. (1998) *La vie des morts: Enquête sur les fantômes d'hier et d'aujourd'hui.* Paris: Imago.

Cardeña, E., Lynn, S.J. and Krippner, S. (eds) (2004) *Varieties of Anomalous Experience: Examining the Scientific Evidence.* Washington, D.C.: American Psychological Association.

Carpenter, M. and Raj, T. (2012) "Editorial introduction: towards a paradigm shift from community care to community development in mental health". *Mental Health and Community Development* 47:4, pp. 457–72.

Carson, R. (1962) *Silent Spring.* Harmondsworth: Penguin.

Carson, R. (1999) *The Edge of the Sea.* London: Penguin.

Carstairs, G.M. (1957) *The Twice-Born: A Study of a Community of High-Caste Hindus.* London: Hogarth Press.

Cassani, C. (2013) "Mental Illness, Addiction and Most Chronic Illness are Linked to Childhood Loss and Trauma". Available at http://beyondmeds.com/2013/12/31/mental-illness-childhood-trauma, accessed on 08 April 2016.

Cassani, M. (2013) "Psychosis, healing and rebirth". Available at http://beyondmeds.com/2013/04/25/psychosis-healing-and-rebirth, accessed 08 April 2016.

CEP (Council for Evidence Based Psychiatry) (2015) "The Maudsley Debate: a cause for hope". Available at http://cepuk.org/2015/05/15/maudsley-debate-cause-hope, accessed on 08 April 2016.

Chapman, C. R. and Gavrin, J. (1993) 'Suffering and its relationship to pain.' *Journal of Palliative Care,* 9, 2, 5–13.

Clarke, I. (2001) *Psychosis and Spirituality: Exploring the New Frontier.* London: Whurr.

Clarke, I. (2010) *Psychosis and Spirituality: Consolidating the New Paradigm.* Chichester: Wiley.

CNWL Equality and Diversity, available at www.cnwl.nhs.uk/about-cnwl/vision-values/equality-and-diversity/, accessed on 12 August 2016.

Cook, C., Powell A. and Sims, A. (eds) (2009) *Spirituality and Psychiatry.* London: Royal College of Psychiatrists.

Cornah, D. (2006) *Impact of Spirituality on Mental Health.* London: Mental Health Foundation.

Cornwell, M. (2012) "I Don't Believe in Mental Illness, Do You?" Available at www.recoverywirral.com/2015/07/alternative-views-on-mental-illness-from-michael-cornwell-ph-d, accessed on 08 April 2016.

Cornwell, M. (2014) "Michael Cornwall Speaks on Helping People in Extreme States with Loving Receptivity". Available at www.youtube.com/watch?v=_Er1bp423Eo&feature=youtu.be, accessed on 08 April 2016.

Council for Evidence Based Psychiatry (2015b) "More Harm Than Good: Confronting the Psychiatric Medication Epidemic". Available at http://cepuk.org/moreharmthangood, accessed on 08 April 2016.

CQC (2011) *Count me in 2010*. London: NMHDU. Available at http://www.cqc.org.uk/sites/default/files/documents/count_me_in_2010_final_tagged.pdf, accessed on 12 August 2016.

Crandell, C. (2014) 'Ireland Investigates Death of 800 Babies at Home for Unwed Mothers". WORLD News Service, 17 June 2014.

Crowley, N. (2006) *Psychosis or Spiritual Emergence? Consideration of the Transpersonal Perspective within Psychiatry*. Essay submitted to Royal College of Psychiatrists SIG.

Davidow, S. (2015) "An Open Letter to Colin Powell". Available at http://www.madinamerica.com/author/sdavidow, accessed on 08 April 2016.

Davies, J. (2014) *Cracked: Why Psychiatry is Doing More Harm Than Good*. London: Icon Books.

de Quincey, C. (2015) "The Philosophy of Panpsychism with Christian de Quincey". Available at www.youtube.com/watch?v=VfevXVQSaNU&feature=youtu.be, accessed on 08 April 2016.

Dewi Rees, W. (1971) "The hallucinations of widowhood". *British Medical Journal* 4:37.DoH (Department of Health) (2005) Delivering race equality in mental health care (DRE), London: DH.

DoH (Department of Health) (2005) *Delivering race equality in mental health care* (DRE), London: DH.

DoH (Department of Health) (2009) *Religion or Belief: A practical guide for the NHS*. London: DH.

Dossey, L. (2001) *Healing Beyond the Body*. Boston, MA: Shambhala.

Dossey, L. (2015) "Consciousness: Why Materialism Fails". Available at http://opensciences.org/blogs/open-sciences-blog/232-consciousness-why-materialism-fails, accessed on 08 April 2016.

Dreger, A. (n.d.) "Shifting the Paradigm of Intersex Treatment, Intersex Society of North America". Available at www.isna.org/compare, accessed on 08 April 2016.

DW (2008) *Film About Thalidomide Victims Breaks Emotional Taboos*. Available at www.dw.com/en/film-about-thalidomide-victims-breaks-emotional-taboos/a-3636886, accessed on 12 August 2016.

Edwards, P. (ed.) (1997) *Immortality*. New York: Prometheus Books.

Ehman, J. (2006) "Studies of Remote Intercessory Prayer: A Bibliography of Articles from the Health Care Literature". Available at www.acperesearch.net/intercessory_prayer_studies.pdf, accessed on 08 April 2016.

Elsaesser-Valarino, E. (2001) *On the Other Side of Life: Exploring the Phenomenon of the Near-Death Experience*. New York: Insight Books.

Esfahani Smith, E. (2014) "A Psychiatrist Who Survived the Holocaust Explains Why Meaningfulness Matters More Than Happiness". *Business Insider*, 22 October 2014.

Evans, M. (1996) "Dying to Help: Moral Questions in Organ Procurement." In D. Dickenson and M. Johnson (eds), *Death, Dying and Bereavement*. Milton Keynes: Open University.

Evans-Pritchard, E. (1940) *The Nuer of the Southern Sudan*. Oxford: Oxford University Press.

Eves, R. (1998) *The Magical Body, Power, Fame and Meaning in a Melanesian Society*. Australia: Harwood Academic Publishers.

Fadiman, A. (2012) *The Spirit Catches You and You Fall Down: A Hmong Child, Her American Doctors, and The Collision of Two Cultures*. New York: Farrar, Strauss and Giroux.

Fenwick, P. and Fenwick, E. (1995) *The Truth in the Light*. London: Headline Book Publishing.

Fenwick, P. and Fenwick, E. (2008) *The Art of Dying*. London: Continuum.

Fenwick, P. and Brayne, S. (2011) "End-of-life experiences: Reaching out for compassion, communication and connection. Meaning of deathbed visions and coincidences". *American Journal of Palliative Care* 28:1.

Fenwick, P. (2012) "Interview on Near Death Experience". Available at www.youtube.com/watch?v=M4PmjKn1zPE, accessed on 08 April 2016.

Fernando, S. (1991) *Mental Health, Race and Culture*. Basingstoke: Macmillan/MIND Publications.

Fernando, S. (2010) "DSM-5 and the psychosis risk syndrome". *Psychosis* 2:3, pp. 196–8.

Fernando, S. (2014) *Mental Health Worldwide: Culture, Globalization and Development*. Basingstoke: Palgrave Macmillan.

Fiore, E. (1995) *The Unquiet Dead*. London: HarperCollins.

Foreign Office (2013) *Forced Marriage*. Available at https://www.gov.uk/guidance/forced-marriage, accessed on 12 August 2016.

Frankl, V. (1983) *The Doctor and the Soul*. London: Vintage.

Frankl, V.E. (2008) *Man's Search for Meaning: An Introduction to Logotherapy*. London: Hodder & Stoughton.

Friedel, D., Schele, L. and Parker, J. (1993) *Maya Cosmos: Three Thousand Years on the Shaman's Path*. New York: William Morrow.

Fuller, C. J. (1992) *The Camphor Flame: Popular Hinduism and Society in India*. Princeton, NJ: Princeton University Press.

Funnell, A. (2014) "Psychiatrists Split on Whether to Ditch DSM". Available at www.abc.net.au/radionational/programs/futuretense/the-psychiatrists-are-revolting/5680842 accessed on 08 April 2016.

Gale, J., Robson, M. and Rapsomatioti, G. (eds) (2014) *Insanity and Divinity: Studies in Psychosis and Spirituality.* London: Routledge.

Gallagher, J. (2015) "Post-Traumatic Stress Evident in 1300BC". BBC News, 24 January 2015.

Geirnaert-Martin, D.C. (1992) *The Woven Land of Laboya: Socio-Cosmic Ideas and Values in West Sumba, Eastern Indonesia.* Leiden: Centre of Non-Western Studies.

Georgatos, G. (2015) "Suicide is heading to a humanitarian crisis – it is a leading cause of death". Available at http://thestringer.com.au/suicide-is-heading-to-a-humanitarian-crisis-it-is-a-leading-cause-of-death-9754#.VtXMj_mLSUk, accessed on 08 April 2016.

Gershom, Y. (1992) *Beyond the Ashes: Cases of Reincarnation from the Holocaust.* Virginia Beach: ARE Press.

Gershom, Y. (1997) *From Ashes to Healing: Mystical Encounters with the Holocaust.* Virginia Beach: ARE Press.

Gidugu, V. *et al.* (2014) "Individual peer support: A qualitative study of mechanisms of its effectiveness". *Community Mental Health Journal* 51:4, pp.445–52.

Good, B. (1994) *Medicine, Rationality and Experience: An Anthropological Perspective.* Cambridge: Cambridge University Press.

Gøtzsche, P. (2014) "Why I think antidepressants cause more harm than good". *The Lancet Psychiatry* 3:2, pp.91–186.

Goulet, J.-G. (1994) "Reincarnation as a Fact of Life among Contemporary Dene Tha." In A. Mills and R. Slobodin (eds), *Amerindian Rebirth.* Toronto: University of Toronto Press.

Goulet, J.-G. (2011) "Understand and manage existential fear: Anthropological approaches to religion and healing rituals". *Ethnologies* 33:1, pp.33–73.

Goulet, J.-G. and Miller, B. (2007) *Extraordinary Anthropology, Transformations in the Field.* Lincoln: University of Nebraska Press.

Goulet, J.-G., Young, D.E. (1994) *Being Changed by Cross-Cultural Encounters: The Anthropology of Extraordinary Experience.* Toronto: University of Toronto Press.

Gray, M. (2011) "Sacred space and the natural world: the shrine of the Virgin Mary at Penrhys". *European Review of History: Revue européenne d'histoire* 18:2, pp.243–60.

Grof, S. (1989) *Spiritual Emergency: When Personal Transformation Becomes a Crisis.* New York: Tarcher Putnam.

Guardian (2015) *Exporting trauma: can the talking cure do more harm than good?* Available at https://www.theguardian.com/global-development-professionals-network/2015/feb/05/mental-health-aid-western-talking-cure-harm-good-humanitarian-anthropologist accessed on 12 August 2016.

Haraldsson, E. (2012) *The Departed Among the Living. An Investigative Study of Afterlife Encounters.* Guildford: White Crow Books.

Hardo, T. (2005) *Children Who Have Lived Before: Reincarnation Today.* London: Rider

Hardy, A. (1997) *The Spiritual Nature of Man: A Study of Contemporary Religious Experience.* Oxford: Oxford University Press.

Haro, J.M. *et al.* (2011) "Cross-national clinical and functional remission rates: Worldwide Schizophrenia Outpatient Health Outcomes (W-SOHO) study". *British Journal of Psychiatry* 199:3, pp.194–201.

Harvey, G. (2002) *Shamanism: A Reader.* London: Routledge.

Heinze, R.I. (1982) *Tham khwan: How to Contain the Essence of Life: A Socio-Psychological Comparison of a Thai Custom.* Singapore: Singapore University Press.

Helman, C. (2000) *Culture, Health and Illness.* London: Hodder Arnold.

Hendry, P., Hill, T., Rosenthal, H. (2014) *Peer Services Toolkit: A Guide to Advancing and Implementing Peer-run Behavioral Health Services.* Albuquerque: ACMHA.

Hickey, P. (2015) *Book Review: Depression Delusion by Terry Lynch,* MD, MA. Available at www.madinamerica.com/2015/08/book-review-depression-delusion-by-terry-lynch-md-ma/, accessed on 12 August 2016.

Horder, J. (2010) "How True is the One-in-Four Mental Health Statistic?" *Guardian,* 24 April 2010.

Houston, T.K. *et al.* (2011) "Culturally appropriate storytelling to improve blood pressure: A randomized trial". *Annals of Internal Medicine* 154:2.

Humphrey, C. (1996) *Shamans and Elders: Experience, Knowledge and Power among the Daur Mongols.* Oxford: Clarendon Press.

Hunter, J. and Luke, D. (2014) *Talking with the Spirits: Ethnographies from Between the Worlds.* Chicago: Daily Grail Publishers.

Hurlbut, H. M. (1992) "Birth practices and infant mortality among the Labuk-Kinabatangan Kadazan of Sabah". *Sabah Society Journal* 9, pp.369–79.

Imperial College (2009) "Unravelling the Mystery of the Self – From Philosophy to Modern Day Science". Available at www.horizonresearch.org/learning-zone/videos-podcasts-2/unraveling-the-mystery-of-the-self-symposium-2009, accessed on 08 April 2016.

Jacobs, S. *et al.* (1997) *Two-Spirit People, Native American Gender Identity, Sexuality, and Spirituality.* Urbana: University of Illinois Press.

Jaspers, K. (1959) *Truth and Symbol: The Apprehension and Consciousness of Being.* London: Rowman & Littlefield.

Joshi, J. (2011) 'Memory transference in organ transplant recipients', *NAMAH 19,* 1.

Kabat-Zinn, J. (2005) *Coming to Our Senses: Healing Ourselves and the World through Mindfulness.* London: Piatkus.

Kaneshiro, N. (2015) "Ambiguous Genitalia". Available at www.nlm.nih.gov/medlineplus/ency/article/003269.htm, accessed on 08 April 2016.

Karter, J. (2015) "Disease Theory of Mental Illness Tied to Pessimism about Recovery". Available at www.madinamerica.com/2015/11/disease-theory-of-mental-illness-tied-to-pessimism-about-recovery, accessed on 08 April 2016.

Kelly, C. and Hooper, D. (2013) "Children's Body Parts Were Kept by Police". BBC News, 22 February 2013.

Kharitidi, O. (1997) *Entering the Circle, Ancient Secrets of Siberian Wisdom Discovered by a Russian Psychiatrist.* London: Harper Collins.

Kinderman, P. (2014) "Why We Need to Abandon the Disease-Model of Mental Health Care". Available at http://blogs.scientificamerican.com/mind-guest-blog/why-we-need-to-abandon-the-disease-model-of-mental-health-care, accessed on 08 April 2016.

Kleinman, A., Eisenberg, L. and Good, B., (1978) "Culture, illness and care". *Annals of Internal Medicine* 88, pp.251–8.

Kleinman, A. (1989) *The Illness Narratives: Suffering, Healing, and the Human Condition.* New York: Basic Books.

Koenig, H. (2007) *Spirituality in Patient Care.* West Conshohocken, PA: Templeton Press.

Krippner, S. (2012) "Spiritually Transformative Experiences". Available at www.youtube.com/watch?v=GOl-zmVl8Tk, accessed on 08 April 2016.

Krippner, S. (2015) "Research perspectives in parapsychology and shamanism". *Paranthropology* 6:1.

Krucoff, M. *et al.* (2005) "Music, imagery, touch, and prayer as adjuncts to interventional cardiac care: the Monitoring and Actualisation of Noetic Trainings (MANTRA) II randomised study". *The Lancet* 366:9481, pp.211–17.

Kübler-Ross, E. (1969) *On Death and Dying.* London: Routledge.

Kübler-Ross, E. (1998) *The Wheel of Life: A Memoir of Living and Dying.* New York: Touchstone.

Kumari, R. (2012) "Confronting India's Culture of Rape". Al Jazeera English, 31 December 2012.

Laderman, C. (1982) *Wives and Midwives: Childbirth and Nutrition in Rural Malaysia.* Los Angeles, CA: University of California Press.

Lenzerini, F. (ed.) (2009) *Reparations for Indigenous Peoples: International and Comparative Perspectives.* Oxford: Oxford University Press.

Levin, J. (2001) *God, Faith and Health: Exploring the Spirituality Healing Connection.* New York: Wiley.

Levine, B. (2015a) "What the Government Knows about Suicide and Depression that We Are Not Being Told". Available at www.madinamerica.com/2015/02/samhsa-knows-suicide-depression-not-told, accessed on 08 April 2016.

Levine, B. (2015b) "Psychiatry's 'Institutional Corruption'". Available at www.madinamerica.com/2015/08/psychiatrys-institutional-corruption-a-chat-with-robert-whitaker-and-lisa-cosgrove, accessed on 08 April 2016.

Lewis, I.M. (1969) "Spirit Possession in Northern Somaliland." In J. Beattie and J. Middleton (eds), *Spirit Mediumship and Society in Africa.* New York: Africana.

Lewis I.M. (2002) *Ecstatic Religion: A Study of Shamanism and Spirit Possession.* London: Routledge.

Lienhardt, G. (1990) *Divinity and Experience: The Religion of the Dinka.* Oxford: Clarendon Press.

Liesowska, A. (2014) "Tattooed 2,500-year-old Siberian Princess 'to be reburied'". *Siberian Times*, 21 August 2014.

Lipton, B. (2014a) "How Does Epigenetics Play a Role in a Developing Infant?" Available at https://biologyofbelief.wordpress.com/2014/08/22/how-does-epigenetics-play-a-role-in-a-developing-infant, accessed on 08 April 2016.

Lipton, B. (2014b) "How Does The Mother's Emotional Well-Being Impact The Child Within Her Womb?" Available at https://biologyofbelief.wordpress.com/2014/11/20/how-does-the-mothers-emotional-well-being-impact-the-child-within-her-womb, accessed 08 April 2016.

Littlewood, R. and Dein, S. (eds) (2001) *Cultural Psychiatry and Medical Anthropology.* New York: Athlone Press.

Longden E., Sampson, M. and Read, J. (2015) "Childhood adversity and psychosis: generalised or specific effects?" *Epidemiology and Psychiatric Sciences* July, pp.1–11.

Longden, E. (2015) "I Hear Voices in my Head, but I'm Fine". *Guardian*, 9 September 2015.

Lucas, C. (2011) *In Case of Spiritual Emergency: Moving Successfully through Your Awakening.* Forres: Findhorn Press.

Luhrmann, T.M. *et al.* (2015) "Differences in voice-hearing experiences of people with psychosis in the USA, India and Ghana". *British Journal of Psychiatry* 206:1, pp.41–4.

Luke, D. (2012) "Altered States of Consciousness, Mental Imagery and Healing." In Simmonds-Moore, C. (ed.), *Exceptional Human Experiences, Health and Mental Health.* Jefferson, NC: McFarland.

Luke, D. (2013) "Psychedelics, Parapsychology and Exceptional Human Experience." In Adams, C. *et al.* (eds), *Breaking Convention: Essays on Psychedelic Consciousness.* London: Strange Attractor Press.

Lukoff, D. (2007) "Visionary spiritual experience". *Southern Medical Journal* 100:6.

Lynch, T. (2015) *Depression Delusion: The Myth of the Brain Chemical Imbalance.* Dublin: Mental Health Publishing.

MacIsaac, T. (2014a) "Psychologist Says Children with Past-Life Memories Exhibit PTSD Symptoms". *Epoch Times*, 1 December 2014.

MacIsaac, T. (2014b) "Near-Death Experiencers Shouldn't Be Treated as Crazy: Healthcare Workers Discuss". *Epoch Times*, 29 August 2014.

Maisel, E. (2011) "What do we mean by 'Normal'?" Available at www.psychologytoday.com/blog/rethinking-psychology/201111/what-do-we-mean-normal, accessed on 08 April 2016.

Malinowski, B. (1929) *The Sexual Life of Savages in North-West Melanesia.* London: Routledge and Kegan Paul.

Manne, R. (ed.) (2001) "In denial: The stolen generations and the right". *Quarterly Essay* 1.

Manning, C. (n.d.) "Interview at the College of Medicine". Available at www.college ofmedicine.org.uk/healthcare-professionals/creative-thinkers-healthcare-professionals-speak/interview-dr-chris-manning, accessed on 08 April 2016.

Manning, C. (2012) "Creating Resilience: Preventing GP Burnout". Available at www.collegeofmedicine.org.uk/healthcare-professionals/reports-reviews/creating-resilience-preventing-gp-burnout, accessed on 08 April 2016.

Manning, C. (2013) "My experience of burnout has led me to help other doctors facing it". Available at www.pulsetoday.co.uk/views/opinion/my-experience-of-burnout-has-led-me-to-help-other-doctors-facing-it/20002801.article, accessed on 08 April 2016.

Margetts, J. (2015) "Woman Reducing Indigenous Suicide Rates through 'Care Factor'; New Program Launched to Tackle Issue". ABC News, 20 August 2015.

Marohn, S. (2014) "What a Shaman Sees in a Mental Hospital". Available at www.wakingtimes.com/2014/08/22/shaman-sees-mental-hospital, accessed on 08 April 2016.

Mate, G., "This Video Dispels Every 'Nature VS Nurture' Myth You've Ever Heard. The Implications are Profound". Available at www.filmsforaction.org/watch/this-video-dispels-every-nature-vs-nurture-myth-youve-ever-heard, accessed on 08 April 2016.

Mate, G. (2014) "It's a Mythology to Think in Terms of Normal & Abnormal". Available at www.youtube.com/watch?v=G-hECo_OB4g, accessed on 08 April 2016.

Matsuura, K. (2001) in K. Stenou (ed) 'UNESCO Universal Declaration on Cultural Diversity', Johannesburg: UNESCO.

McCaffrey, A. et al. (2004) "Prayer for health concerns, results of a national survey on prevalence and patterns of use". Archives of Internal Medicine 164:8, pp.858–62.

McGrath, J. et al. (2015) "Psychotic experiences in the general population". JAMA Psychiatry 72:7, pp.697–705.

McKee, L. (2016) "Suicide of the Ceasefire Babies". Available at http://mosaicscience.com/story/conflict-suicide-northern-ireland, accessed on 08 April 2016.

McLaren, N. (2013) "What's wrong with psychiatry explained by a psychiatrist". Available at www.youtube.com/watch?v=f3kJ0nA6gNw&feature=share, accessed on 08 April 2016.

McNay, I. (2012) "Interview with Dr Peter Fenwick 'Consciousness and Dying'". Available at http://consciouslifenews.com/dr-peter-fenwick-consciousness-dying-interview-iain-mcnay/1127410, accessed on 08 April 2016.

McNeill, D. and Coonan, C. (2006) "Japanese flock to China for organ transplants". The Asia Pacific Journal. Available at http://apjjf.org/-David-McNeill/1818/article.html, accessed on 08 April 2016.

Metzl, J.M. (2010) The Protest Psychosis: How Schizophrenia Became a Black Disease. Boston, MA: Beacon Press.

Metzl, J. (2014) "The Protest Psychosis: Race, Stigma, and the Diagnosis of Schizophrenia". Lecture at Durham University, 4 April 2014.

Miller, P. (2015) *EMDR for Schizophrenia and Other Psychoses*. New York: Springer Publishing.

Mills, A. (1994) "Nightmares in western children: An alternative interpretation suggested by data in three cases". *Journal of the American Society for Psychical Research 88,* pp.309–25.

Mills, A. and Slobodin, R. (1994) *Amerindian Rebirth: Reincarnation Belief among North American Indians and Inuit.* Toronto: University of Toronto Press.

Mind (2007) "Putting the South back into Psychiatry". Available at www.mind.org.uk/media/192444/mindthink_report_1.pdf, accessed on 08 April 2016 .

Miovic, M. (2009) "The relevance of non-local studies to health". *NAMAH: Journal of Integral Health* 17:3.

Mitchell, S. (2015) "Another Albino Child Is Murdered and Mutilated in Tanzania". *Vice News,* 15 February 2015.

du Monchaux, P.-J (1766) "Anecdotes de Médecine". Lille: J.B.Henry *Imprimerie.*

Moncrieff, J. (2009) *The Myth of the Chemical Cure: A Critique of Psychiatric Drug Treatment.* Basingstoke: Palgrave Macmillan.

Morehouse, D. (2000) *Psychic Warrior: True Story of the CIA's Paranormal Espionage Programme.* West Hoathly: Clairview Books.

Morgan, J. (2003) 'Spirituality.' *Bryant 03-I-vol-I,* 112. Available at www.uk.sagepub.com/upm-data/5235_Bryant_Spirituality.pdf, accessed on 12 August 2016.

Mottram, K. (2014) *Mend the Gap: A Transformative Journey from Deep Despair to Spiritual Awakening.* Gorleston: Rethink.

Nandi, J. and Ghosal, A. (2012) "This Silent Protest Heard Loud And Clear". *The Times of India,* 30 December 2012.

Nasr, S.H. (1996) *Religion and the Order of Nature.* Oxford: Oxford University Press.

NHS England (2014) *Actions for End of Life Care: 2014–16.* Available at https://www.england.nhs.uk/wp-content/uploads/2014/11/actions-eolc.pdf, accessed on 12 August 2016.

NIH (National Institute of Health) (2015) *Team-based treatment is better for first episode psychosis.* Available at www.nimh.nih.gov/news, accessed on 08 April 2016.

NIMHE (2001) *Inspiring Hope,* NIMHE National Project on Spirituality in Mental Health, in partnership with The Mental Health Foundation.

Nelson, J. (1994) *Healing the Split.* Albany, NY: State University of New York Press.

Nerlich, A.G. *et al.* (2000) "Ancient Egyptian prosthesis of the big toe". *The Lancet* 356:9248, pp.2176–9.

Norton, K. (2007) "A brief history of prosthetics". *InMotion* 17:7, pp.11–13.

Nygren-Krug, H. (2001) *Health and Freedom from Discrimination.* Geneva: World Health Organization, Publication Series, No. 2. Available at www.who.int/hhr/activities/q_and_a/Health_and_Freedom_from_Discrimination_English.pdf, accessed on 08 April 2016.

Obeyesekere, G. (1981) *Medusa's Hair: An Essay of Personal Symbols and Religious Experience.* Chicago: University of Chicago Press.

O'Neil, S. (2015) "Knowing How Doctors Die Can Change End-Of-Life Discussions". Available at www.npr.org/sections/health-shots/2015/07/06/413691959/knowing-how-doctors-die-can-change-end-of-life-discussions, accessed on 08 April 2016.

Osis, K. (1961) *Deathbed Observations by Physicians and Nurses.* New York: Parapsychology Foundation.

Parker, C. (2014) "Hallucinatory 'Voices' Shaped by Local Culture, Stanford Anthropologist Says". Stanford News Report, 16 July 2014.

Parnia, S. (2007) *What Happens When We Die.* London: Hay Publishing.

Parnia S. *et al.* (2014) "AWARE-AWAreness during resuscitation – a prospective study". *Resuscitation* 85:12, pp.1799–1805.

Parry, J. (1994) *Death in Banares.* Cambridge: Cambridge University Press.

Passi V (2011) *Excellence in Medical Education Issue 1.* AoME, Academy of Medical Educators.

Paton, M. (2012) "Sin and the Single Mother: The History of Lone Parenthood". *Independent,* 25 May 2012.

Pearsall, P. (1998) *The Heart's Code,* London: Thorsons.

Périgaud, L. (2012) *"Entre IL et ailes".* Available at www.entreiletailes.com/wp-content/uploads/2012/04/Press-kit_Between-Two-Spirit.pdf, accessed on 08 April 2016.

Pick, A. (2015) "Auschwitz, Memory and Truth: How Trauma Passes down the Generations", *Guardian,* 27 June 2015.

Polimeni, J. (2012) *Shamans among us: Schizophrenia, Shamanism and the Evolutionary Origins of Religion.* Lulu.com.

Pollack, S. (2012) "The Magdalene Laundries: Irish Report Exposes a National Shame". *Time,* 7 February 2013.

Polson, J. and Mackovic, B. (2006) *The Implantable Artificial Heart Project, press release.* Available at www.heartpioneers.com/releases/090506.html, accessed on 12 August 2016.

Puchalski, C. (2001) "The role of spirituality in health care". *Proceedings of Baylor University Medical Centre* 14:4, pp.352–7.

Quinn, M. (2004) "The Complete Marbles, exhibition". Available at http://marcquinn.com/exhibitions/solo-exhibitions/the-complete-marbles, accessed on 08 April 2016.

Radin, D. (2016) "Selected Peer-Reviewed Psi Research Publications". Available at http://eanradin.com/evidence/evidence.htm, accessed on 08 April 2016.

Rael, J. (2012) *Being and Vibration.* North Carolina: Millichap Books.

Ramos, D. (2014) "Interview". Available at http://crazywisefilm.com/2014/11/17/interview-dagmar-ramos-spiritist-psychiatrist, accessed on 08 April 2016.

Rankin, M. (2005) "An introduction to religious experience". RERC Third Series, Occasional Paper 2.

RawOrg (2011) "The End of Delivering Race Equality." Available at www.mind.org. uk/media/273467/the-end-of-delivering-race-equality.pdf, accessed on 08 April 2016.

Razzaque, R. (2014) *Breaking Down is Waking Up: Can Psychological Suffering be a Spiritual Gateway?* London: Watkins Publishing.

Read, J. (ed.) (2004) *Models of Madness: Psychological, Social and Biological Approaches to Schizophrenia.* London: Routledge.

Read, J. (2015) "Interview". Available at http://crazywisefilm.com/2015/04/22/ john-read-maoris-viewpoint-on-hearing-voices, accessed on 08 April 2016.

Redbridge Faith Forum (n.d.) "To Comfort Always". Available at http://mylife. redbridge.gov.uk/uploadedFiles/Redbridge/Redbridge_Homepage/zMyLife_ redesign/Categories/Difficult_times/To%20Comfort%20Always.pdf, accessed on 08 April 2016.

Reichel-Dolmatoff, G. (1997) *Rainforest Shamans.* Totnes: Themis Books.

Rhodes, J.E. *et al.* (2016) "A qualitative study of refugees with psychotic symptoms. Psychosis: Psychological, social and integrative approaches". *Psychosis* 8.1.

Ring, K. (2008) *Mindsight: Near-Death and Out-of-Body Experiences in the Blind.* Bloomington, IN: iUniverse Press.

Roberts, Y. (2013) "Forced Adoption: The Mothers Fighting to Find their Lost Children". *Guardian*, 27 October 2013.

Roe, C.A., Sonnex, C. and Roxburgh, E.C. (2015) "Noncontact healing: What does the research tell us?" *European Journal of Integral Medicine* 7:6, pp. 687. 1876–3820.

Romme, M. and Escher, S. (1993) *Accepting Voices.* London: Mind.

Romme, M. (2011) *Psychosis as a Personal Crisis.* London: Routledge.

Rosenhan, D.L. (1973) "On being sane in insane places". *Science* 179:4070, pp.250–8.

Rosenthal, P.A., and Rosenthal, S. (1980) "Holocaust effect in the third generation: child of another time". *American Journal of Psychotherapy* 34:4, pp.572–80.

Russell, D. (2015) "How a West African Shaman Helped my Schizophrenic Son in a way Western Medicine Couldn't". *Washington Post*, 24 March 2015.

Rutherford, L. (2008) *The View through the Medicine Wheel: Shamanic Maps of How the Universe Works.* Shrewsbury: O Books.

Sabom, M. (1998) *Light and Death*, Grand Rapids: Zondervan.

Saleha, R.T. (n.d.) "Customs of Death in Pakistani Culture". Available at www. Academia .Edu/6257624/CUSTOMS_OF_DEATH_IN_PAKISTANI_ CULTURE, accessed on 08 April 2016.

Saine, A. (2004) *Teachings: Psychiatric Patients, Pure Classical Homoeopathy.* Noida: B. Jain.

Sartori, P. (2008) *Near-Death Experiences of Hospitalized Intensive Care Patients: A Five Year Clinical Study*. Lewiston, Queenston, Lampeter: Edwin Mellen Press.

Schlitz, M., Wiseman, R., Watt, C. and Radin, D. (2006) "Of two minds: Skeptic-proponent collaboration within parapsychology". *British Journal of Psychology* 97:3, pp. 313–22.

Schultz, W. (2015) "The chemical imbalance hypothesis: an evaluation of the evidence". *Ethical Human Psychology and Psychiatry* 17:1.

Scull, A. (2015) *Madness in Civilisation: A Cultural History of Insanity*. London: Thames & Hudson.

Seikkula, J. (2011) *Psychosis: Psychological, Social and Integrative Approaches, The Comprehensive Open-Dialogue Approach in Western Lapland*: Routledge.

Seikkula, J. *et al.* (2006) "Five-year experience of first-episode nonaffective psychosis in open-dialogue approach: Treatment principles, follow-up outcomes, and two case studies". *Psychotherapy Research* 16:2, pp.214–28.

Seikkula, J. *et al.* (2011), "The comprehensive open-dialogue approach in western lapland: ii. Long-term stability of acute psychosis outcomes in advanced community care". *Psychosis* 3:3, pp.192–204.

Shahar, Y. (2014) *A Damaged Mirror: A Story of Memory and Redemption*. Alfei Menashe: Kasva Press.

Sheldrake, R. (2013) "The Science Delusion, Banned Ted Talk". Available at www.youtube.com/watch?v=JKHUaNAxsTg&feature=youtu.be, accessed on 08 April 2016.

Sherwood, H. (2016) "Anglican Church Risks Global Schism over Homosexuality". *Guardian*, 12 January 2016.

Shulevitz, J. (2014) "The Science of Suffering. Kids Are Inheriting Their Parents' Trauma. Can Science Stop it?" Available at https://newrepublic.com/article/120144/trauma-genetic-scientists-say-parents-are-passing-ptsd-kids, accessed on 08 April 2016.

Smith, A. *et al.* (2012) "Risk of cancer in first seven years after metal-on-metal hip replacement compared with other bearings and general population". *British Medical Journal*. Available at www.bmj.com/content/344/bmj.e2383, accessed on 08 April 2016

Smith, R. (2000) "A good death", *British Medical Journal* 320:7228, pp.129–30.

Somé, M.P. (1995) *Of Water and the Spirit: Ritual, Magic and Initiation in the Life of an African Shaman*. Harmondsworth: Penguin.

Sprangers, M. and Schwartz, C. (1999) "Integrating response shift into health-related quality of life research". *Social Science and Medicine* 48:11, pp.1507–15.

Sri Aurobindo, (1970) *Letters on Yoga*, vol.1:8, 431. Available at www.sriaurobindoashram.org/ashram/sriauro/downloadpdf.php?id=41, accessed on 08 April 2016.

Stein, R. (2006) "Researchers Look at Prayer and Healing". *Washington Post*, 24 March 2006.

Stevenson, I. (1977) "The Southeast Asian interpretation of gender dysphoria: An illustrative case report". *Journal of Nervous & Mental Disease* 165:3.

Stevenson, I. (1997) *Where Reincarnation and Biology Intersect*. Westport, CT and London: Praeger.

Stockmann, T. (2015) "The UK National Health Service Peer-Supported Open Dialogue Project". Available at www.madinamerica.com/2015/10/the-uk-national-health-service-peer-supported-open-dialogue-project, accessed on 08 April 2016.

Szasz, T. (2010) *The Myth of Mental Illness*. London: Harper Perennial.

Taleb, N.N. (2010) *The Black Swan: The Impact of the Highly Improbable* (2nd ed.). London: Penguin.

Tart, C. (1997) *Body, Mind, Spirit*. Charlottesville, VA: Hampton Roads Publishing.

Tart, C. (2011) "Reincarnation Overview". Available at http://blog.paradigm-sys.com/reincarnation-overview, accessed on 08 April 2016.

Tart, C. (2015) "Interview with Parapsychological Association". Available at www.youtube.com/watch?v=MBIO5eH3u-Q&feature=share, accessed on 08 April 2016.

Taylor, L.M. (2000) "Saving face: acid attack laws after the UN convention on the elimination of all forms of discrimination against women". *Georgia Journal of International & Comparative Law* 29, pp.395–419.

Taylor, S. (2016) "Breakdowns and 'shift-ups'. The relationship between psychosis and spiritual awakening". *Psychology Today*, 12 February 2016.

Thich Nhat Hanh (1999) *The Miracle of Mindfulness: An Introduction to the Practice of Meditation*. Boston, MA: Beacon Press.

Thich Nhat Hanh (2014) *No Mud, No Lotus: The Art of Transforming Suffering*. Berkeley, CA: Parallax Press.

Thomas, P. (2014) *Psychiatry in Context: Experience, Meaning and Communities*. Ross-on-Wye: PCCS Books.

Thomas, P. (2015) *Madness in Civilisation: A Cultural History of Insanity*. Available at www.madinamerica.com/2015/04/madness-civilisation-cultural-history-insanity, accessed on 08 April 2016.

Thomson, H. (2015) "Study of Holocaust Survivors Finds Trauma Passed on to Children's Genes". *Guardian*, 21 August 2015.

Tobert, N. (2000) "Mystical, Spiritual and Religious Experiences: An Exploration of the Relationship between Spiritual Experience and Mental Health". Dissertation for MSc in Medical Anthropology, Brunel University.

Tobert, N. (2001) "Consciousness and health: Another perspective from India". *Network: Scientific and Medical Network Review* 75.

Tobert, N. (2007) "In-Sanity: explanatory models for religious experience". Occasional Paper 3, Series 3, RERC: Religious Experience Research Centre.

Tobert, N. (2008) *Mental Health Needs Assessment with Black and Minority Ethnic (BME) Communities*. Harrow: Harrow Primary Care Trust.

Tobert, N. (2010a) *Bridging Cultures, Dissolving Barriers, Mental Health Promotion with BME Communities, End of Year Evaluation Report 2009/2010*. Harrow: NHS Harrow.

Tobert, N. (2010b) *Somali Advocacy Research Report.* Available at www.aethos.org.uk/research, accessed on 08 April 2016.

Tobert, N. (2014) *Spiritual Psychiatries: Mental Health Practices in India and UK.* CreateSpace Independent Publishing Platform.

Tobert, N. (2015a) "Shamans and Psychiatrists, a Comparison". Available at www.madinamerica.com/2015/01/shamans-psychiatrists-comparison, accessed on 08 April 2016.

Tobert, N. (2015b) "Human Experiences in Academic Boxes". Available at www.madinamerica.com/2015/01/human-experiences-academic-boxes, accessed on 08 April 2016.

Tobert, N. (2016) "Knowledge frameworks in medicine and health". *NAMAH: Journal for Integral Health* 23:4.

Tolle, E. (n.d.) "Awaken to a Life of Purpose and Presence". Available at www.eckharttolletv.com/s/2fgvfl, accessed on 08 April 2016.

Topping, A. (2014) "NHS Mental Health Care in Crisis". *Guardian,* 8 October 2014.

Truth and Reconciliation Commission of Canada (2015) *Honouring the Truth, Reconciling for the Future Summary of the Final Report.* Available at www.trc.ca/websites/trcinstitution/index.php?p=905, accessed 08 April 2016.

Turner, V. (1967) *The Forest of Symbols: Aspects of Ndembu Ritual.* Ithaca, NY: Cornell University Press.

Van Gordon, W., Shonin, E., Griffiths, M. (2016) *Are contemporary mindfulness-based interventions unethical?* BJGP.

Van Lommel, P. (2011) *Consciousness Beyond Life, The Science of the Near-Death Experience.* London: Harper Collins.

Van Lommel, P. *et al.* (2001) "Near-Death experience in survivors of cardiac arrest: A prospective study in the Netherlands". *The Lancet* 358: 9298, pp.2039–45.

van Os, J. and Kapur, S. (2009) "Schizophrenia", *The Lancet* 374:9690, pp.635–45.

Vige, M. *et al.* (2009) *A Challenge For The Mental Health Professions.* Mind Think Report 4.

Villoldo, A. (2015a) "Interview". Available at www.youtube.com/watch?v=to2mQrfZ W1Y&sns=fb, accessed on 08 April 2016.

Villoldo, A. (2015b) *One Spirit Medicine: Ancient Ways to Ultimate Wellness.* London: Hay House.

Walker, D. (2015) "Quantitative Mental Health & Oppression, Part Two: The Case of the 'American Indian'". Available at www.madinamerica.com/2015/02/quantitative-mental-health-oppression-part-two-case-american-indian, accessed on 08 April 2016.

Wardle, E. (2014) "Death in the Consulting Room: Memories of the Holocaust and Questions of Past Lives". MA thesis, Middlesex University.

Watters, E. (2010) *Crazy Like Us: The Globalization of the American Psyche.* New York: Simon&Schuster.

Weiner, A. (1976) *Women of Value, Men of Renown: New Perspectives in Trobriand Exchange.* Oxford: Wiley.

Whitaker, R. (2010) *Anatomy of an Epidemic.* New York: Broadway Books.

Whitaker, R. (2015) "Psychiatry through the Lens of Institutional Corruption". Available at www.madinamerica.com/2015/05/psychiatry-through-the-lens-of-institutional-corruption, accessed on 08 April 2016.

Whitaker, R. and Cosgrove, L. (2015) *Psychiatry under the Influence, Institutional Corruption, Social Injury, and Prescriptions for Reform.* New York: Palgrave Macmillan

WHO (2001) "Mental Disorders Affect One in Four People". Available at www.who.int/whr/2001/media_centre/press_release/en, accessed on 08 April 2016.

WHO (2016) "Female Genital Mutilation". Available at www.who.int/mediacentre/factsheets/fs241/en, accessed on 08 April 2016.

Williams, W. and Johnson, T. (2015) *Two Spirits: A Story of Life With The Navajo.* Maple Shade, NJ: Lethe Press.

Winkelmann, A. and Güldner, F.H. (2004) "Cadavers as teachers: the dissecting room experience in Thailand". *British Medical Journal* 18:329(7480), pp.1455–7.

Woo-kyoung, A., Proctor, C., and Flanagan, E. (2009) "Mental health clinicians' beliefs about biological, psychological, and environmental bases of mental disorders". *Cognitive Science* 33:2, pp.147–82.

Yehuda, R. *et al.* (2015) "Holocaust Exposure Induced Intergenerational Effects on *FKBP5* Methylation". *Biological Psychiatry.* Available at www.biologicalpsychiatryjournal.com/article/S0006-3223(15)00652-6/abstract, accessed on 08 April 2016.

Yehuda, R., Golier, J. and Kaufman, S. (2005). "Circadian rhythm of salivary cortisol in Holocaust Survivors with and without PTSD". *American Journal of Psychiatry* 162, pp.998–1000.

Yehuda, R. (2015) "How Trauma and Resilience Cross Generations". Available at www.youtube.com/watch?v=LXgZamuTe3Q, accessed on 08 April 2016.

Yock, T.I. *et al.* (2016) "Long-Term Toxic Effects of Proton Radiotherapy for Paediatric Medulloblastoma". *The Lancet Oncology.* Available at www.thelancet.com/journals/lanonc/article/PIIS1470-2045(15)00167-9/abstract, accessed on 08 April 2016.

Young, D.E., Goulet, J.G., (1994) *Being Changed: The Anthropology of Extraordinary Experience.* Toronto: University of Toronto Press.

Zamperetti, N. *et al.* (2003) "Defining death in non-heart beating organ donors". *Journal of Medical Ethics* 29, pp.182–5.

Zessin, D. (2015) *Codex Alternus: A Research Collection of Alternative and Complementary Treatments for Schizophrenia, Bipolar Disorder and Associated Drug-Induced Side Effects.* Omaha, NE: Alternative Communications Publisher.

Zutshi, V. (2012) "The Stargate Project: Psychic Warriors and the CIA". Available at http://realitysandwich.com/158056/stargate_psychic_warriors_cia, accessed on 08 April 2016.

SUBJECT INDEX

AUTHOR INDEX

Natalie Tobert, PhD, is a medical anthropologist who has done original research in India, Sudan and the UK. She has been leading workshops and training on different cultural understandings of health for the past twenty years. Natalie lives in London.